THE WARRIOR WELLBEING TOOLKIT

SELF HELP TOOLS AND TECHNIQUES TO AWAKEN YOUR INNER WARRIOR AND LIVE A LIFE OF WELLBEING AND HAPPINESS

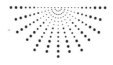

CAROL-ANN REID

authors
AND CO.

CONTENTS

CAROL-ANN REID

WELLBEING WARRIOR TOOL KIT

*E*very 40 seconds someone loses their life to suicide...

Approximately 1 in 4 people in the UK will experience a Mental Health problem each year.

1 in 6 people report experiencing a common mental health problem (such as anxiety and depression) in any given week.

1 in 5 people experience mental health issues without ever being diagnosed.

75% of people with diagnosable mental health conditions receive no treatment at all.

Mental illness is the largest single burden of disease in the UK.

Mental health issues are responsible for 91 million workdays lost in the UK. These issues in the workplace cost about £30 billion per year.

The cost of mental health issues to the economy (£105 billion) is similar to the entire budget of the NHS.

Suicide is the most common cause of death for men aged 20-49.

(MHFA England statistics)

Those 40 seconds ticked right on by as you were reading those heart-breaking statistics. It is time for us to not only raise more awareness around mental health and wellbeing, but to get proactive and learn what it takes to be a Wellbeing Warrior.

I have loved and lost someone incredibly close to me to suicide. There is nothing in life that can prepare you for that type of heartbreak and the tsunami of emotions that follow. I have struggled with anxiety in the past and felt my confidence and self-belief drop to the floor many times. I work alongside people who have lost hope and come from a place of surviving rather than thriving.

I grew up in the most loving, supportive home but saw people struggle to live with depression, with no professional support or guidance beyond medication and a sick note slapped into their hands. They were left with no choice but to paint the war paint on and try to make it through the day, sometimes not for themselves, but for those that they loved unconditionally.

If you are going through your own mental health and wellbeing journey; I honour you, I see you, I feel you. You are not alone.

This book has been created to bring us together in unity. The Warriors you are about to discover are here to help shed light where there may be darkness, and empower you with their wisdom, expert knowledge, skills, and tried and tested techniques that you can introduce into your own life. They have each, like me, been in the trenches.

They have felt first-hand what it is like to live with the fear of what the future may hold, not knowing if or when the dark clouds will lift. In their own unique ways, they have worked through their struggles to establish a healthier relationship with their mental health and cultivate their wellbeing.

But let me share something with you before you delve into this book; their struggles have made them into Warriors. I have called upon this tribe of Wellbeing Warriors to share their expert advice and teachings to help guide you to take your own physical, mental and spiritual health back into your own hands.

I have now worked in the mental health, wellbeing and mindset arena professionally for the best part of a decade, but I have been a Wellbeing Warrior in the making all my life, and every trial and tribulation has taught me great lessons - greater lessons than any university degree could have.

From a young age I have always been an observer and empath, I despised seeing others in pain. Both my parents worked, and still do, for the NHS. Their jobs are to support people's physical health, which is incredibly important and inspiring. But I have always felt a gap between the support that is available for physical health and mental health.

If you break a bone, you get whisked away to A&E and are treated immediately, but what if you are paralysed by social anxiety or depression? What if you are going through a tough period in your life and your confidence and self-worth has hit rock bottom?

I have been working on a 1-2-1 coaching basis with clients, both adults and even children, many who have slipped through the net, been put on a 6-8 month waiting list to speak to a counsellor and if their symptoms persist and they agree, be medicated to suppress the feelings and emotions they are experiencing due to ill mental health and wellbeing.

Before I continue, a heartfelt disclaimer; I am not a medical professional and I always advise that you seek medical help, should you need to. I do support the use of prescription medication to support mental health and wellbeing.

But what I wish to bring into the world through the Warrior movement and this book is an additional set of tools to aid us; a toolkit of self-help techniques and strategies that we can each use on a daily basis to help prevent the harrowing statistics rising.

Together we are pushing for a world where proactivity and prevention is taken just as seriously as reactive action and seeking cures.

Clients I have worked with in coaching sessions and workshops have experienced an incredible 360* turn around in their wellbeing from us co-creating a self-help toolkit that they can carry with them wherever they go. They have a set of techniques and methods at their fingertips that they can utilise whenever needed.

This is incredibly empowering because it allows them to take responsibility for their own wellbeing.

The result?

They take their health and happiness back into their own hands, giving them hope, confidence and belief in themselves and their future.

So, where do we start?

Let's start by recognising that there isn't a 'one size fit's all' approach when it comes to mental health and wellbeing. In fact, I believe this is where a lot of the problems stem from.

We live in a society where we are urged to fit in a box and be like other people. Albeit, it is natural for us to want to be a part of tribe, it's in our DNA, but when it comes to nurturing our individual health and mental wellbeing, we must be brave enough to step outside of the box and discover what best suits us as individuals, not just go off what worked for a friend or colleague and dismiss everything else.

Or worse, give up on yourself if something doesn't work the first-time round. We are each as individual as our fingerprints, with a completely unique mind, body and spirit. This is why I knew this book had to be a collaboration.

It is filled with lessons and self-help advice from 15 individual experts in wellbeing. Warriors who have been through incredibly tough times themselves and are sharing their collective wisdom.

Take from it what resonates with you.

Over the years, I have created my own warrior wellbeing toolkit. It's invisible to the eye but inside lies magic.

When I decided enough was enough and I couldn't continue feeling how I was, I made a promise to myself to be open minded to alternative therapies, treatments and even the spiritual side of healing. When you reach rock bottom, you are willing to try anything, right?!

My friends and family thought I was losing the plot

when I tried describing a Kinesiology session I had, and they switched off after I mentioned crystals and energy healing. When I came home with a rubber band on my wrist after investing in life coaching and CBT (Cognitive Behavioural Therapy), I was met with 'what's that rubber band meant to do'?

When the non-spiritual people in my life questioned my belief in the power of NLP (Neuro Linguistic Programming) and my decision to spend time in London getting my NLP Master Practitioner qualification, I simply told them it was 'Wizardry School for the mind'.

By then I had become quite resilient to the raised eyebrows I got, because I could feel the internal shift that was happening as a result of learning these new tools and methods, and that was what was important to me.

And now? People want to know exactly what I do to have such an unshakable mindset, because they can see the changes that have happened as a result.

Since working on my mental health, mindset and wellbeing, I have experienced some incredible life events, that rewind 10 years ago, I never imagined possible for 'little old me'.

I now run my own successful coaching and training business, publishing my second book, have a radio show called 'Feel Good Friday' been featured on podcasts and in magazines as a 'mindset expert', worked alongside large organisations welcoming the Warrior Wellbeing into the workplace, married the love of my life, have a tribe of warriors around me who I can truly call friends, finally made peace with my body and self-image, and after trying for a baby for 6 years, I can now say we are expecting as I write this.

It's only when you connect the dots looking back do you fully recognise how much of an impact your mindset and wellbeing has on your life. I used to say 'I could never write a book or be a speaker, I'm dyslexic', this belief paralysed the dreams I had, until I changed that internal story and belief to 'I can do anything I put my mind to'. Another example is I used to say for many years 'I bet I'm not able to get pregnant', from there my cycles stopped and my body felt the full effect from my worry and stress. The last year I have focused on changing that belief, nurturing my body and like magic, we are now being blessed with not one baby, but two! Yes, I'm sure you can imagine the beautiful shock we had when we were told we had two little twin Warriors on the way!

Had I have not had a shift in my mindset and made my wellbeing a priority, all of the above would have still been a distant dream. It's taken hard work, persistency and a ton of courage, but without the initial decision to make a change internally; mentally, physically and spiritually, my life would be very different to what it is today.

One piece of advice when it comes to trying to new

things and worrying about the opinion of others; what other people think of you is none of your business. Find what works for you. That is your primary focus from now on.

Over the years I have reflected on my journey many times, as it's safe to say I have made some monumental hiccups in the past. Everything from relationships with dangerous people to careers that were not aligned with who I was, lying to loved ones, cheating on others and falling into a dangerous 'rock and roll' lifestyle.

Each and every path I took lead to a dead end where I'd feel empty, unfulfilled and trapped. I didn't know which way to turn, never mind who to turn to. So, I stuck to what I knew; I'd dust myself off and simply carry on, choosing to blame the world for my problems.

At that time, I would swear I didn't know what to do to change how I was feeling or the circumstances I was in. I was a victim to my circumstances. I felt that life was happing to me, rather than for me.

But between me and you, deep down, I knew exactly what I should do to change it.

Instead I ignored my intuition, stayed comfortable being uncomfortable and dismissed the red flags that were warning me things must change!

These red flags would show up as anxiety, IBS, stress headaches, loss of appetite followed by emotional binge eating, tightness in my neck, not wanting to socialise and talking to myself like a bully.

I was so busy being busy, trying my hardest to fit in, be liked by others and follow the crowd that I lost who I was and fell victim to society's cycle of ill-being.

Mortality Motivation

It took me to experience a hattrick of painful life events to say, "THIS IS IT, NO MORE". Something had to change. I call this 'mortality motivation'. So many of us sleepwalk our way through life and over time, we become accustomed to feeling down and anxious and settle for what is.

Until one day, you are hit with a wake-up call that shakes you to your core and shifts your entire perception on life.

Whether it's a near death experience, an illness, loss of a loved one, a relationship or something that creates a change in your life that is out of your control. These things physically make you look at yourself and your life differently. Mortality motivation is life's way of holding up a mirror and saying "look, life is short and incredibly precious. DO NOT waste another day settling for what is. You are worthy of more!"

We all hear the stories of those who get saved from a burning building then go on to quit their job, loose 35lbs, become motivational speakers, live on a boat and adopt 3 kids. As incredibly inspiring as these stories are, you don't need an audacious life changing experience to embark on your own journey of self-improvement and wellbeing. At any point, you can look in the mirror and decide to take your future into your own hands

What triggers this tidal wave of change for people is a shift in their perception of what is important. They have an inner knowing that life is short and in order to grow and evolve, they must take responsibility and make it happen themselves. The penny drops. They awaken.

I want to empower you to make changes in your life before mortality motivation strikes.

Every single day is an opportunity to stop, check in with yourself and ask yourself some honest questions and decide from there what your next steps are.

Here are some questions that can help you become more self-aware:

Am I OK?

How am I feeling today?

Is how I am feeling effecting my physical or mental health?

Am I making choices that support my wellbeing and future?

Do I need support or guidance through anything?

Whether you answered yes or no to the above questions,

they have now given you something incredibly powerful; the power of choice.

Do you choose to carry on regardless, hoping that one day, something will change?

Or do you choose to look at what your options are and make some different decisions:

Do you choose to seek support?

Do you choose to take action?

Do you choose to do things differently?

Do you choose wellbeing or illbeing?

I began asking myself these questions on a regular basis. Depending on my answer, I would either give myself a pat on the back for feeling good and on track with my mindset, or I would hypothetically look in my warrior toolkit and choose to take something from it that I knew would help me to feel better and more empowered.

Worrier V's Warrior thinking

In 2005, the National Science Foundation published an article regarding research about human thoughts per day. The average person has around 50,000 - 70,000 thoughts per day. Of those, the research evidenced that around 80% of those thoughts are negative and 90% are habitual, meaning they are the same repetitive thoughts day in, day out.

These studies reveal that the quality of our wellbeing rests on the quality of our internal and external communication. It also reveals how our bodies respond to the way we think, feel and act. This is often called the "mind-body-spirit connection". When we feel guilt and shame or stress and anxiety, our bodies cry out to tell us that something isn't right. For example, high blood pressure, a headache or a stomach ulcer might develop after a particularly stressful event. Therefore, it is crucial to learn how to raise your self-awareness and tune into your mind, body and spirit.

So, if 90% of our thoughts are habitual, and up to 80% of them are negative, where does this leave us in terms of changing the way we think?

I for one tried for many years just 'thinking positively' but it never helped me get to any root cause of the negativity or anxiety, nor did it last long term.

This is where I came across CBT and I've since trained thousands on how the model works, and how to implement this powerful way of thinking into everyday life.

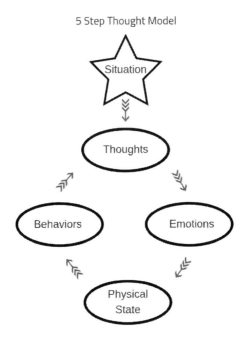

Diagram: The CBT Mindset Model

What this demonstrates is that your thoughts influence your emotions, your emotions effect your physical state, which in turn effect your behaviours, which then loops back around and influences your thoughts.

Here's an example; The situation is you have a job interview coming up, the thoughts you have racing around in your mind are 'what if I fail', and 'I just know I'm not going to get the job, there are so many other more qualified people going for it'.

How do you think these thoughts will affect your emotions? You may feel anxious, apprehensive, nervous, worried, worthless, upset.

How do you think these emotions will affect your physical state? You may be shaky, clumsy, sweaty, have a headache or stomach-ache.

What will your behaviours be like as a result of this? You may find yourself pacing around, being short and snappy with those around you, you may even pull out of the interview.

Your thoughts as a result of these behaviours? 'I knew I would end up messing this up', or 'who am I to think I could go for this job'.

And the cycle continues.

I call this the 'worrier' way of thinking. Where your thoughts go straight for the negative or you worry about what may or may not even happen. This way of thinking will have a direct effect on your mental and physical health and will impact many experiences you go through in life.

Now imagine if you were to approach the job interview with what I call 'Warrior' thoughts.

If you were to think 'I've got this', or 'I will give it my everything and that is the best I can do', how do you think your emotions would be affected? You may feel empowered, excited, possibly a little nervous as it is natural to feel so in some situations, but all in all your emotions would be much more neutral. As a result of these emotions, now imagine what your physical state and behaviours may be?

You may be focused, calm and able to prepare for the interview much better and all in all have a clearer mind and balanced physiology.

Can you see the huge difference between the 'worrier' thinking and the 'warrior' thinking? Imagine the impact the different ways of thinking have on the results you will see. Yet the scenario, i.e. the job interview, is the same for both the worrier and the warrior. The warrior way of thinking is empowering, impactful and much more productive in terms getting the desired result.

When you work on changing your worrier thoughts to warrior thoughts, you have greater self-awareness and your resilience is strengthened as a result.

You begin to see things from a different perspective. You're able to face life's challenges with a more resilient mindset and your mental, physical and spiritual health dramatically improves as a result.

Are you a worrier or warrior?

What is your go-to way of thinking?

Ask yourself these questions and answer them to yourself

honestly. Anyone, and I mean anyone no matter what age, background, gender, race, experience can change their thinking from that of a Worrier to a Warrior.

Now I'm going to share with you the most powerful tool that I personally used when I first began my recovery from being a serial Worrier, and what helped me evolve into the Warrior I am today. It is so powerful in fact that I have spent the last few years creating a physical self-help tool, that is now available online for adults and children to buy.

That is the Awakening the Warrior CBT Band.

It stemmed from a CBT technique and is known as the gold standard approach to therapy by the NHS.

How it works:

You start by placing the Warrior band on your non dominant wrist, it acts as a trigger for you to become self-aware, each time you look at the band you pause for a moment and ask yourself 'what am I saying to myself in my mind?' or 'what am I thinking?'

If it is something negative, or it is the worrier self-talk, you simply recognise it, give your band a gentle 'snap' and then replace the thought with a Warrior thought; something more positive. You continue to repeat this process every time you catch yourself having those worrier thoughts.

So, the 3 'R Steps' to remember are:

1. Recognise

2. Replace

3. Repeat

How does this work?

What I love about this CBT technique is it is simple but incredibly effective. The science behind it is fascinating and enough to turn any raised eyebrows into raving band fans (speaking from experience here!)

The band firstly acts as a trigger for you to become more aware of your self-talk and how you are feeling, the snap of the band interrupts the thoughts, causing the thought patterns in your brain to break as a result. This is the key! Once you have interrupted the chatter and snapped out of the unconscious mind and re-entered the conscious mind, this gives you a window of opportunity to purposely replace the old thought with a new one of your choice.

The result?

Over time and with practice, the band becomes not only a trigger for you to check in with yourself, but it becomes an empowering 'anchor' that every time you wear your band, it makes you feel powerful and in control of your thoughts and feelings. It anchors in your feeling of being a Warrior along with all the associated thoughts you have practiced and imprinted into your belief system. Clever right?

When you change your thoughts, you will change your life. Your thoughts affect your emotions and your emotions affect your behaviour. Break this habitual cycle and replace unwanted thoughts with positive and empowering Warrior thoughts and you will change your emotions and behaviours as a result.

Your thoughts create your reality.

Here are some examples of common worrier thoughts:

I'm not good enough.

What if I fail?

What will people think of me?

I can't do this.

Here are some examples of Warrior thoughts you can choose to replace them with:

I am good enough.

I will try my hardest.

What people think of me is none of my business.

I can do this this.

What can the Warrior band be used for?

Overcoming anxiety and worrier thinking.

Changing old habits and forming new empowering ones.

Quitting smoking.

Fear of flying.

Nerves around public speaking.

You can begin to create your own list of Warrior mantras and affirmations, and you can find a range of Warrior resources, including the bands on the website shared at the end of this chapter to help you take yourself from being a Worrier to a Warrior once and for all.

As you progress through the rest of the book and meet your fellow wellbeing warriors, you may notice a common thread that runs throughout their personal journeys and the lessons and tools they share with you. That is, that at some point along their journey, they have all Awakened their inner Warrior, and discovered the 'Warrior Code' in their own unique way.

The A-E Warrior Code is this:

Awareness

Belief

Courage

Discipline

Evolve

Through my journey and awakening, I discovered there is a code we can follow that guides us from a place of ill-being to wellbeing. From anxious to aligned. From darkness to light.

Here is a breakdown of the Warrior Code:

A - The first step of following the Warrior Code is to become self-aware. Without self-awareness, you have very little platform to build your wellbeing on. When you become aware of how you are feeling physically, you begin noticing what feels good and what doesn't. You then have the power to recognise if your thoughts are worry-based and causing anxiety, or Warrior based and empowering. Then there is of course being aware of how you feel spiritually. This means checking in with your energy, are you feeling high energy and high vibration? Or are you feeling low energy and low vibration? Also, when you become more aware of how you feel spiritually, it helps bridge the gap between the mind and body. You get to recognise when you feel in flow and overall more harmonious. Becoming more self-aware is the first step to taking responsibility for where you are in life. From here, you can start to change anything about it.

B – The second step is belief; having belief in yourself and being open to believing that there is a greater energy (source, universe, guidance, higher self, God). When you believe in yourself, you unlock power from within. You release limiting beliefs that may have held you prisoner to the past and kept you playing small in the world. Self-belief is your very own superpower; no one else can give it to you. You may have had people say to you 'I believe in you', yet it still wasn't enough for you to break through your own internal barriers and step into your personal power.

When you are open to believing that there is a greater energy surrounding you, protecting you, guiding you by giving you signs and support, this is when you open yourself up to another level of wellbeing, health and happiness. If you haven't read or watched 'The Secret', this is a great starting point to connecting and believing in the laws of the universe and how energy impacts our lives.

C – Courage is like a muscle, the more courageous action we take, the stronger we get. We are all born with confidence and courage, if you watch a young child play in the park you will see true bravery and courage as they leap off swings, wave at other children and even strangers. It's through conditioning over the years that we are told to 'stay safe' and 'don't do that', where we get our lights dimmed and begin to play it safe in life. But to truly step into your Warrior power and practice living a life of wellbeing, you may have to do things that are out of your comfort zone. You can take a breath, tell yourself you are brave and take courageous action. Whether it's trying out a new fitness class, saying 'no thank you', to that extra glass of wine or saying yes to an exciting opportunity. Courage comes from within; courage lies within you right now.

D – Discipline is a hurdle that many fall at, but not you, Warrior! New research by Phillipa Lally, a health psychology researcher at University College London, revealed it takes an average of 66 days to form a new habit. The 21-day myth has been debunked. Knowledge is power. Now you know that it takes an average of 2 months for a habit to be formed, the discipline becomes less daunting. It's a case of integrating your wellbeing into your daily routine until it becomes a part of your everyday lifestyle and who you are. Consistency is key when it comes to your wellbeing.

E – You are on a never-ending journey of self-discovery and improvement. When you acknowledge this fact, you can accept yourself as you are at this present moment in time, at this particular point in your journey. You are evolving into the happiest, healthiest version of you. Just as the world around you is evolving, it takes time and patience. It's important that you stop and celebrate yourself along the way. In doing so, you get a chance to look back and see how far you have come. This is an exciting opportunity to see your own personal evolution unfolding!

My wish is that you enjoy and embrace the diversity and courage that this book entails. My hope is that you take from it what resonates with you and create your very own Warrior wellbeing toolkit by trying out the exercises and expert advice shared. My request is that you join the Warrior movement and help spread this book and message far and wide.

Love and light, Carol-Ann.

AUTHOR BIO

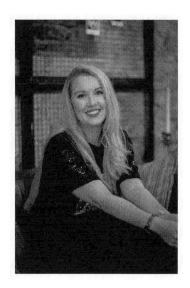

Carol-Ann is the founder of the Awaken the Warrior movement. She is an Intuitive Life Coach, Master NLP Practitioner and CBT Coach, Speaker, Trainer and Best Selling Author, based in the North West.

Having battled her own metal health struggles and loosing a loved one to suicide, Carol-Ann is on a heart-led mission to empower people become more resilient and fulfilled through giving them the self-help tools and techniques they need to support their own mental health and wellbeing.

She has worked alongside companies including RedBull and Emmaus UK delivering talks and workshops around Mental Health and Warrior Wellbeing in the Workplace, sharing her unique teachings and skills.

Carol-Ann and her team of wellbeing warriors are incredibly passionate about bringing mental health and wellbeing support into companies and organisations.

Carol-Ann has been featured in magazines such as B1 and Liberty, she has been interviewed as a guest on numerous podcasts including Jairek Robbins' highly acclaimed 'What The World Needs More Of' and hosts her own radio show called 'Feel Good Friday'.

She has a gift for helping people overcome their inner challenges, discover who they truly are and awaken their inner Warrior.

You can find many supportive free resources, meditation downloads and more information about the Awaken the Warrior CBT bands by visiting Carol-Ann's website: www.carolannreid.com.

You can also find more information about working with Carol-Ann as a coach or enquire about workshops and talks on the website.

Where to connect with Carol-Ann:

LinkedIn: Carol-Ann Reid

Facebook support group: Awaken the Warrior Within

facebook.com/carolannreidcoach

instagram.com/carolannreidcoach

2

ALICE LYONS

LESSONS IN SELF EXPRESSION

*M*y four-year-old self gave precisely zero fucks what anyone thought of her.

I constantly bubbled with energy that I'd throw into whatever outlet I could find. Finger-painted 'artworks' covered every surface in the house. I invented games to inflict on my two sisters and would fly into a passionate rage if they dared to object. I spouted endless streams of waffle at my parents, never letting a minute pass without having another random thought which I *had* to share.

"Everybody stop and listen to me!"

"Do we have a choice, Alice?"

"No."

Truth be told, I was a total pain in the arse. But I was nothing if not expressive. It served me well. I was a very happy child, and, despite all the noise, people did find my bolshie nature entertaining.

The thing about being an expressive child is that you need to be kept occupied. All the time.

My parents sent me to a different club every night of the week and all-day on a Saturday. In my mind, they were rewarding me for doing so well in school. On reflection, they were looking for a break. It was a source of great relief to them that I would always look to talk with anyone I met out in public.

They could get some much needed 'quiet time' by letting me wander off to make new friends. (Don't worry - it was the nineties. Nothing bad ever happened in the nineties.)

When I was six years old, we visited a family activity centre where a particularly grumpy pottery instructor selected me to assist him with a demonstration. Unbeknown to him, I was a *talker*.

As I took my place at the wheel in front of a crowd of children and parents, I immediately launched into an unsolicited origin story of how I came to be there that day, pointing out my family and explaining why my brother wasn't with us that day.

"He doesn't always come out with us because he's a lot older than the rest of us, so he doesn't like doing kids' stuff. He has a different dad and he lives with him in a different

part of Bristol. His dad's name is Steve. He's ok, but he always smells of smoke, and..."

The potter cut me off abruptly. *"Alright kid, I didn't ask to hear about your family tree"*. He rolled his eyes in exasperation and my cheeks started to flush as the onlookers chuckled.

I felt myself die a little inside. I was used to having a captive audience who engaged with my nonsensical musings. Now I was faced with a critic, I didn't know how to deal with it.

To the potter, it was a throwaway comment sparked by a minor irritation that was probably forgotten within a day. But to me, I'd committed a crime. My story had caused so much upset to this man that public humiliation had been necessary to put me in my place.

Lesson 1: Not everyone wants to hear your opinion. Ironically, they can be very vocal about this.

That was the first time I fully understood the idea that not everyone cares for your opinion. To a friendly, people-loving child, this was a harrowing realisation.

I internalised the guilt of having upset this stranger and

turned it into a personal attack on my character. I made a problematic assumption – *you can hurt people with your words, so maybe it's better to keep your opinions to yourself. That way, people will like you more.*

It's funny how small, random experiences in our childhood can affect us years into the future. But the more evidence I found to support this world view, the more I began to intentionally hold myself back.

As I moved through secondary school, my desire to be liked outweighed my desire to be myself. I found myself dumbing down my personality to fit in with a questionable friendship group. I found myself becoming quieter, less funny, less outspoken and less engaging to avoid being teased or criticised for my honest opinions.

In essence, I learnt to become less than myself.

Lesson 2: Choosing not to express yourself means choosing self-censorship.

As I found myself increasingly restricted at school, my outlet became my home. My parents continued to encourage my outspoken nature, and this manifested in ever more energetic ways. I became argumentative and we'd get into screaming rows where I'd throw all my frustrations at my mum in a full-frontal assault.

It was unwarranted and unfair, but I couldn't help myself.

As children and young adults, we don't have the self-awareness or emotional intelligence to be able to question our behaviour. We don't usually look at ourselves objectively and question the motivation behind our actions. We are emotional time bombs, which will go off under the right (or wrong) circumstances.

My emotional outbursts were damaging my relationship with my parents. But in school, emotional repression seemed to be serving me well.

Teachers loved how compliant I was in lessons. My 'friends' enjoyed having me in their group as a 'yes girl' to laugh along with their jokes and make them look good. All evidence pointed to the fact that towing the line was beneficial.

I was rewarded with the very thing I always wanted; I was well liked. I had a wide social circle and got on with everybody to a comfortable degree.

What a life. Nobody had a bad word to say about me and I maintained this perpetual popularity into my early adulthood. Life was very much ok.

Very much ok.

Unequivocally, categorically.... just *ok*.

* * *

After the end of another busy shift in the coffee shop, I arrived at my bus stop in the deserted business district and collapsed onto the bench. My feet throbbed. The familiar stench of stale coffee seeped through my crumpled jumper. 9pm. Late again. Another 15 hour shift down. Same again tomorrow.

How was this my life? Six months earlier I'd graduated from uni with a respectable degree after doing everything I was told to do for the past ten years. I'd passed all the exams, followed the school-college-uni trajectory and kept any thoughts of deviancy to myself.

Where was the fast-track graduate scheme I'd been promised?

What did I have to show for the years of hard work?

A minimum wage management position, working 60 hours a week.

My eyes drifted lazily to the office block on the opposite side of the road. I could see the security guard sitting behind the marble reception desk, bathed in the soft, warm golden glow of the halo-shaped light fixture.

Not for the first time, I imagined what it would be like to work in that office.

I imagined my heels clacking as I walked across the

polished stone floors of the reception. I'd smile at the guard as he'd buzzed me through the security gate.

I imagined the mirrored doors of the lift sliding open, ready to take me to the top floor.

I saw the comforting green light over the emergency exit door leading me out of the building.

I felt the cool hit of the air wash over me as I stepped onto the rooftop.

The familiar crunch of gravel as I walked over to the edge.

I'd spend a few quiet moments taking in the view of the city I grew up in. A few silent goodbyes to the places I had loved and hated over the past 23 years.

And then, I'd jump.

I half-smiled through the tears that had gathered while I played through this scenario. It was a comforting fantasy I replayed on an increasingly regular basis. However bad, mediocre or indifferent my day had been, it was reassuring to know that there would always be a way out if I wanted to take it.

It would be another six years before I would share these suicidal thoughts with anyone.

I'd go through therapy, a long process of personal development, further education and two relationships before acknowledging the fact that I'd felt suicidal, off and on, throughout my twenties. I hadn't just hidden the truth from the people closest to me. I had hidden it from myself.

Lesson 3: Self-censorship can become so natural to us that it becomes invisible.

'Self-expression' can sound ridiculously hedonistic. To me, it used to conjure images of self-important artists making extravagant artworks. To a girl who had dimmed so much to fit in, it was something abstract, out-of-reach and bordering on intimidating.

But over the past few years, I've changed my stance on this, significantly.

To me, self-expression is the key to true personal wellbeing. Being able to express ourselves honestly helps us develop a deeper and healthier connection with who we *actually* are, versus who we *think* we should be.

It was only when I realised that I had been suppressing my personality for most of my life that I discovered the life-changing power of self-expression. I remembered that gutsy, fire-cracker of a child who didn't care what anybody thought of her, or her outspoken opinions or terrible paintings, thank you very much. She was truly herself, in all her glory, at all times.

The thing is, she didn't disappear overnight.

In fact, she never really disappeared at all. She just became obscured by layers of social conditioning that told her to be somebody different for the benefit of other people.

Social conditioning is the process by which we are encouraged to fall into particular and 'acceptable' patterns of behaviour based on societal norms. It's particularly influential and insidious because, much like self-censorship, it can be invisible to us.

The world is presented to us in a certain way as we go about our lives, from the lessons we are taught in school to the news we watch on tv to the content we consume on social media. Because we receive these messages every day, they become normalised to us, and so we can easily adopt the same world view that our native society holds because it feels natural to do so.

Lesson 4: Readily adopting society's world view can mean radically dismissing our own.

I first learnt about this social conditioning in college

during media studies. My teacher, Ned, was one of the most brazen and out-spoken grown-ups I had ever met in the education system. He swore often, and always told us the truth, whether we wanted to hear it or not. I liked him immediately.

He'd launch into passionate rants to try and convince us that the images we saw on our screens weren't as real as we believed them to be.

"Just because something is non-fiction, doesn't make it true", he'd say. *"See that image? It's been constructed. A cameraman chose where to stand, he's framed this shot using his knowledge of composition, he's chosen when to pan to a revealing shot. He's holding the camera without a stabilizer, so it looks gritty and shitty so that we interpret it as 'real'. It's all done to get you to feel something specific. It's been constructed".*

I felt a wave of despondency wash over me. I reluctantly put my hand up to ask a grim question:

"If everything we see in the media is a lie, how can we believe anything we see?"

He cocked his head and sighed a little. It was no secret that Ned genuinely cared about his students, and he wanted us all to be well armed before heading out into the big bad world.

"My girl, just because it's not all true doesn't mean it's a lie. There's a difference".

He could read the confusion on my face. He continued.

"Everything we see is a version of the truth – it's some-body's representation of their truth, but we need to indi-vidually decide if it matches with our version. We don't need to be told what to believe by other people, and if people are presenting things as factual, it's up to us to question them using our own judgement".

Lesson 5: Acknowledging other people's views is important. Expressing our own is vital.

This bombshell came at the right time. I had recently recognised the need to socialise with people who were more on my wavelength, and my newfound friends were giving me the confidence to be myself and share my real thoughts. I revelled in my expressive course subjects, delighting in art, design, theatre production and, most of all, writing.

Ever since learning to write, I had obsessively poured my time into creating stories, penning my own books with illustrations alongside - complete with a blurb and barcode written on the back cover.

I wrote two sequels to Aladdin years before Disney ever made the films. Annoyingly, I didn't have the foresight to copyright them.

As a teenager, I started voraciously journaling.

My journal got the full brunt of every uncomfortable, embarrassing or unsettling thought I ever had. It was the place I could dissect the days as they happened to try to make sense of them all. There was also a lot of moaning about boys. A ridiculous amount. I dread to think about all the tears and ink wasted.

Therein lay the problem with my teenage journaling style; it was purely reflective.

More often than not, I'd be looking *back* on things that had already happened. Very rarely would I think about the future or my aspirations for it. I would never set goals or expectations beyond a few weeks.

I might ruminate about how I'd like a particular scenario to end, but I didn't think about the bigger picture of what this would mean for my life. I didn't have dreams. I didn't have a vision.

This is one of the reasons my mental health deteriorated rapidly through my twenties. Depressive episodes and suicidal thoughts began creeping in around the age of 19 and would visit ever more frequently as I struggled to find my place in the world.

During a messy work-experience-cum-gap-year, I would go for long drives across the country thinking about when and where I would steer my car off the road.

It was a terrifying time because I didn't know who to talk to about these suicidal thoughts, or why they were happening.

I had everything to be grateful for; a good family, awesome friends, bags of potential – everything that should make me happy and successful.

But it all felt hollow. Meaningless. Directionless.

Lesson 6: Holding back our darker thoughts gives them a firmer hold over us.

I decided to start a public speaking course last year on a bit of a whim. I didn't have any reason to do it. It wasn't a prerequisite for my job in interior design, and I had no aversion to doing presentations, pitches or talks on demand if I had to. But I felt oddly compelled to do it.

Three months of rave reviews and excellent feedback later, I was approaching the final stretch of the course, but I suddenly felt that I wasn't pushing myself as much as I should be.

My peers were having to overcome phenomenal hurdles, challenging themselves to speak in English as their second language, or overcoming terrific stage fright in order to present. Meanwhile I was sticking to cute and fluffy crowd-pleasing topics which I knew would guarantee a warm reaction from the crowd. I was just about to waste a golden opportunity.

I looked to my favourite Ted Talks for some inspiration, and the answer was glaringly obvious to me. The common thread which ran through all of them was to approach a deeply personal, taboo or traumatic subject matter but deliver it with heart, humour and bravery. The best talks challenged the audience as much as the speaker and united them all in facing down the danger together.

That was what I needed to do.

One evening, I dared myself to talk about the most uncomfortable subject I could think of and fell asleep hoping I would wake up with the answer as to what it would be.

That night I dreamt I was learning to sail a flagship. An elderly Captain hurriedly gave the basics before abandoning ship, bellowing 'She's all yours now, good luck!'

It hardly seemed acceptable to be putting so many lives at risk. As I looked across the deck at the faces of the crew, I suddenly realised 'holy shit, this is your boat now – do something!'

We set off without incident and seemed to be making good progress while the weather was inclement. But then a storm rolled in.

The crew did the best they could to keep the boat afloat, but without instruction from me, their efforts were scatty, disjointed and ineffective. Waves tore across the deck, throwing dozens of people into the sea, myself among them.

When I surfaced, I was a long way from the ship, surrounded by dark water. I felt a visceral terror as I fought against the waves to make the arduous journey back.

As the dream-hours passed, I was faced with a decision; I could continue with the struggle, or I could stop and let myself drown.

I understood the metaphor completely. It was a reflection of my thoughts around suicide.

'Alright', I conceded when I woke up. 'I get the hint'.

Lesson 7: Our intuition is our subconscious mind expressing itself freely
----

A week later, I had re-written my speech and was preparing to present at the end of the course. For the first time, my classmates could see I was truly nervous. My palms sweated as I went between choosing to deliver my new 'Dark Water' speech or retreating to previous iterations about community engagement. Something less suicide-y. I still hadn't decided if I had the guts for this.

I thought about my parents in the audience who had no idea what I was about to tell them. You think you know your kid completely after 30 years. Surprise!

I delivered 'Dark Water' with a lump in my throat the whole way through. It was the single most terrifying but liberating experience of my adult life. An incredible amount of power comes from speaking the whole truth after a decade of repression, it's hard to qualify with words. All I can say is that I recommend it.

After leaving the stage, the next speaker rushed up to give me a hug. "I know how you feel, I've seen the dark water as well", she whispered. I burst into tears. *Vindication.*

At the end of the event, a swathe of people approached me to congratulate me on the speech, but the striking thing was their willingness to share so many of their own experiences. I was shocked by how many people had shared similar feelings and how deeply they had resonated with my story.

It solidified in me a desire to keep talking. I felt like the cork had been pulled from a bottle and there was no containing it again. It felt too important.

Lesson 8: When you express yourself freely, you send out a call to other likeminded people

----

A few weeks later, I released the first episode of my podcast series. 'Dark Coffee' starts unfiltered conversations around mental health and wellbeing in an attempt to normalise these topics.

My mission is to create safe spaces to have brave, open and connecting conversations which let other people know that, however they're feeling, their feelings are valid, they matter, and they are never alone with them.

Over the time I've been producing the podcast, it has become my go-to method for self-expression. Being able to put words to complex emotions has given me the headspace to process them on a deeper level, giving my brain a chance to calm the fuck down.

Often when we're emotionally distressed, our brains will race into overdrive or slow to a crawl. When I have felt my thoughts become foggy, I have picked up a microphone to talk myself round to clarity.

One such incident gained notoriety in my community; an episode which was fittingly titled 'Depression in Real Time'. Publishing the episode was terrifying but, much like my speech, I believed that voicing my dark, scary thoughts would help someone else shed light on their own experience.

The biggest lesson I've learned about self-expression is that, so often, it's not just about you. It's about using your own experience as a way of reaching out to others, to draw a line of connection between previously disparate parties and say 'Hey, I see you. I feel the same way. You're not that weird, I promise'.

Lesson 9: Self-expression is not just about you. It's about drawing a line of connection with others.

OK, there's an even bigger lesson. As with every area of personal growth and character development, self-expression is a *practice*. I talk, train and educate around mental health every day and still struggle to talk about my experiences with my own parents.

We're not all going to be comfortable expressing ourselves 100% honestly 100% of the time and, honestly, I think that's a good thing.

Our desire to fit into our social groups is part of our survival instinct and it would feel counterintuitive to ditch it completely.

There's nothing wrong with wanting to be liked, and I've learnt to accept that needy, childlike part of myself that wants to be friends with everyone. My inner child is basically a puppy. I think it's endearing.

So, for you, dear reader (you bloody lovely thing) I leave you with my parting lesson:

Lesson 10: Self-expression is a practice, so find an outlet you enjoy and keep trying.

Ideas for Practicing Healthy Self-Expression:

- Create a 'vision board' – an electronic or physical collage of your future goals.
- Write a letter to someone you need to express strong sentiments towards (probably best not to send it! That way, you can be brutally honest).
- Use the voice recording feature on your phone to record a 'stream-of-consciousness' to empty the thoughts out of your head.
- Dance naked in the rain.... Too much? Alright, maybe put some music on when you first wake up and dance yourself awake.
- Write about your top 5 values to help you discover what's important to you.
- Challenge yourself to have one uncomfortable

conversation every day to develop the habit of airing minor grievances at the point where they are easily manageable.

- Post an 'unfiltered' social media post, letting people see you as you really are with an honest and expressive caption to match.

- Start a daily journaling habit – have a look online for journal prompts if you need a few ideas. A great start is to write 3 things you are grateful for in the morning, along with one thing you'd like to achieve that day, and then write a summary sentence in the evening about what you've achieved, learned or experienced.

- Make a group decision in a social situation; choose the film you'll watch, the restaurant you'll eat in or the route you'll walk.

- If someone says something that you don't agree with, be respectful of their opinion, but challenge it. Fiercely and unapologetically.

AUTHOR BIO

ALICE LYONS

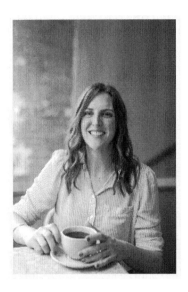

Alice Lyons is a mental health speaker, podcaster, writer and trainer based in Manchester.

She is the Founder and Director of 'Dark Coffee' – a wellbeing company which starts unfiltered conversations around mental health.

The aim is to normalise subjects from suicide to self-esteem and empower individuals, organisations and communities to develop a proactive and receptive mental health culture.

Alice is an active member of the Manchester business community and produces video content and articles on Linked In to help mission-led business owners develop the skills to be able to express themselves authentically and promote their services effectively.

She recently co-produced and presented a documentary around suicide prevention which will be released in the Autumn of 2019. The *Dark Coffee* podcast is available through all major streaming services.

Contact:

Email: talk@darkcoffee.co.uk

LinkedIn: linkedin.com/in/alicelyons

Podcast: Dark Coffee

instagram.com/alice.lyons.wellbeing

3

ALLISON ROSE

THE REVOLVING DOOR OF ANXIETY

*W*hen a kid uses a revolving door, they smile with joy and excitement. They're in awe they can go round and round without having to get out. Even when dizzy, they'll push it a few more times running in circles and giggling. They're in the moment, not considering what others might think. It's pure enjoyment.

In some ways anxiety is like being stuck in a revolving door, but not some fancy one at a swanky hotel. I'm talking about an old rundown one that creaks and sticks – no fun at all.

Doubting, negative self-talk had me spinning in circles and never seemed to dissipate. It didn't end with just one question, such as "what if I say the wrong thing?" I would come up with an answer to it, rethink my answer, create another one, ruminate on that for awhile, and ultimately conjure up a few more questions. I felt compelled to follow that circular process and struggled with that for the majority of my life. There was no moving forward.

The plan for this chapter is to share with you the journey I've had with social anxiety. This will include a few examples of my life struggles, helpful and unhelpful coping skills, and what ultimately encouraged me to make changes. Following that, I will share my goal for telling my story and some tips that have helped guide me to where I am today.

It all started when I was a kid, worrying about absolutely everything. At this age I struggled more with generalized anxiety compared to social anxiety, with my first memory of it being as far back as six years old. I remember scribbling on a small 3x3 white piece of paper "I love you," followed by two X's and lines where my parents could sign, as if it were a contract affirming their love for me.

I also recall worrying about a multitude of other things, such as the possibility of a tornado when it was windy outside or that my parents would get a divorce when they were having a disagreement. In addition, I recall refusing to leave my mom's side at stores, following so close behind that I often stepped on the back of her shoes. Naturally my mom was frustrated by that and encouraged me to look at something in another aisle, to no avail. I was too scared to wander off. "What if I couldn't find her again? I'd be lost forever." Just to be clear, I knew my parents loved me, I've never seen a tornado, my parents haven't gotten a divorce, and I've never been lost - well at least not for long. There was no validity to my worries. Later in life, to my amazement, I learned these issues seemed nonexistent to others and didn't even cross their mind; however, my anxiety took these outwardly insignificant issues and amplified them to the point they became all-consuming. Why was my "normal" so different than everyone else's? Why did I think about things so differently than others did and obsess over them until I felt stuck? It was exhausting.

For the time being, though, I assumed everyone else felt and thought the same way. I didn't know any different, and how could I? I was just a kid. But because of that, I didn't address it with my parents, and the lack of overt red flags made it challenging for them to recognize there was an issue. Parents aren't mind readers. They would've done anything in their power to help if they only knew, but I didn't even know. I wasn't able to identify that the butterflies in my stomach were the result of anxiety and was unaware that what I was experiencing or feeling even had a name. It's difficult to determine whether I would've been able to comprehend what anxiety meant even if someone tried explaining it to me.

As I grew older, I began struggling more with social anxiety and the debilitating fears of how people were evaluating me. It didn't matter if it was a complete stranger or my best friend I had known for years. It was always in the back of my head that I would be judged and found lacking.

Public speaking of any sort was a challenge. Irrational thoughts raced through my mind, exponentially increasing any doubts. "You're going to mess up. You're going to forget everything. You're going to turn bright red. Everyone's going to stare at you and laugh." Repeating these negative thoughts was a chain reaction, leading to the physiological symptoms. My face turned bright red, my chest became heavy and tight while my heart raced, and I talked a mile a minute. I also despised playing "popcorn" in class, which is a game when a student reads a portion of a chapter aloud and then calls on a classmate to proceed with the next section. I rarely understood the material because I was too busy silently reading ahead, trying to prepare myself in case I was called on. Both of these examples represent occasions I had convinced myself that my peers would be critical of me, and their standards were unattainable. The mental representation I constructed of how I thought my peers viewed me, as well as their expectations, were not based in reality. I say that because I received good grades, and I was never criticized by my peers. There wasn't any evidence to back up my beliefs.

During my school years, I lacked confidence and was incredibly shy. "Allie, speak up. We can't hear you." It became annoying constantly hearing that, and you'd think I would have learned to simply speak up after being told that countless times. Nope, not me. Someone once told me that the shyness and lack of confidence people exhibit can be a smokescreen for anxiety – a place to hide. I suppose that's why I never started speaking up. Anxiety was the underlying issue, and each time I was called on, negative self-talk and worry overcame me. "Why would I want someone to hear my answer? What if it was wrong?" To clarify, lack of confidence and shyness does not indicate anyone's intelligence. I managed to do quite well in school.

The list of what I struggled with goes on and on, but fortunately for me, I discovered an outlet for the anxiety when I was a teenager. I had participated in gymnastics recreationally, but it wasn't until I began competing and spending numerous hours in the gym that I noticed the benefits. The anxiety turned into an asset, as I channeled my nerves, worries, and fears into energy that became a driving force at the gym. Any emotional energy that had built up during the day I expended through physical activity. Furthermore, because the sport requires immense concentration, it gave me something temporary to focus on instead of ruminating. For instance, rather than scrutinizing a conversation with a friend, wondering why she was ignoring me and somehow concluding I had said something wrong, I was focused on my routines and skills. The anxiety was finally manageable and least noticeable during this time, but unfortunately it was short-lived due to an injury.

After getting injured, it was the emotional pain not the chronic pain that eventually broke me. I lost a major part of my identity and one of the only places I felt comfortable expressing myself. It's difficult for me to fully understand why I wasn't incapacitated by the anxiety when in gymnastics. Even though I competed individually on each apparatus, I also competed as part of a team, which may have been a contributing factor. My teammates didn't judge me or make me feel inferior for falling or for missing a skill. They were always encouraging, understanding, and loving. I didn't recognize the amount of support and acceptance I felt by being a part of a team until it was gone. I felt completely lost without the structure of being at the gym, being a part of a team, and the ability to creatively express myself. Without having an outlet for my anxiety, the symptoms returned full force. I was desperate to find something that would ameliorate the symptoms and help me find acceptance and friends elsewhere. Drinking was the norm at my school and seemed like an easy way to solve all my problems.

When I lost gymnastics, I turned to something unhelpful – alcohol – to try to manage the difficult thoughts and feelings I continued to experience and to discover a place of acceptance. Alcohol gave me an out, a short-term release from the anxiety that I gladly welcomed. It seemed like the perfect way to drown out the thoughts, and to be honest, I enjoyed it. Because alcohol decreases inhibitions, I felt free, a completely new experience for me. This was the first time I didn't wonder if people were judging me, I didn't calculate my every move, and I basically didn't care. In a way it was liberating – I was finally able to socialize without analyzing everything and feeling scared. I wasn't debilitated by fear and made a lot of new friends. But it was still a revolving door, not really going anywhere.

Maladaptive coping skills, like drinking, are only a temporary relief. The stressor – in this case, my anxiety – either remains constant or increases in intensity. It's like putting a band-aid over a wound, making it feel better for the moment. It merely masks the anxiety. I realized what I was doing was not healthy, so I cut down on alcohol in order to focus on college. But as a consequence of decreasing my alcohol consumption, my symptoms once again returned with full intensity and reclaimed the reigns all the way into my 20s.

It's not particularly enjoyable for me to think about my 20s because I wasted a large portion of those years limiting myself. I declined a number of activities and experiences because I was afraid of failing and also worried how people would view me. The entire time I was simply judging myself, and to be honest, people probably didn't care what I was doing or wouldn't have even noticed. In many ways, anxiety is not about other people; it's about the intrapersonal conflict within oneself. There's a constant internal monologue that demands attention. It came to the point where I was no longer dating and barely spending time with friends. My life consisted of attending school and working with my social life being essentially nonexistent.

Watching on the sideline as my friends started getting married, having kids, and purchasing their first homes was an eye-opener for me. At 28 (soon to be 29), the big 3-0 was around the corner, and I too, wanted all of those things. But how did I expect to get married or have children when I was too intimidated to even date?

It's ironic because the anticipation of turning 30 was ultimately what encouraged me to make changes. It felt like a major milestone in my life, and if I didn't make some sort of change now, I doubted I ever would. Living life the way I was did not seem feasible because I wasn't really living. I was simply existing. It took me awhile to realize this, but if I wanted change, I was the person that needed to do it and to put forth the effort. As much as I wanted my mom to swoop in and save me, she couldn't help this time. No one could. I realized this entire time I had been using anxiety as a crutch, a way to justify I wasn't capable of doing certain things, but anxiety wasn't holding me back. I was.

Some days I prayed it would merely disappear, so I wouldn't have to face it. The first step was allowing myself to feel afraid because avoiding it, over time, had become habitual and felt safe. But it's okay to feel scared and vulnerable. Actually, it's quite healthy. "Feel the fear and just do it anyway" became my mantra. I was in control, and I always had been. I just didn't know it.

Don't get me wrong, there are still plenty of things I'm working on, and I still experience anxiety on a daily basis. My family and friends can certainly vouch for that. There's no easy fix or pill to take that will cure it because it's a lifelong journey. It deserves tune ups just like any car does. It doesn't completely disappear; it just becomes more manageable, giving me the opportunity to engage in more enjoyable activities. It's not the anxiety that has changed – I have. I changed my relationship with it, and that has made all the difference. My new way of thinking has led to new actions, and I've shared these with you at the end of this chapter.

It's incredible to reminisce over the past year or so, acknowledging I have tried more things in that short time than I have in the last five years. For me, these accomplishments are worthy of celebration. The highlights include traveling for the first time solo, starting to date again, meeting new friends, and sharing this story. Two years ago, I would've never imagined that I'd have been on multiple dates within a few months or met a new friend by sharing a table with her and deciding to exchange numbers. That used to be unheard of for me. I was the person with my head down hoping people would just walk on by without noticing. In the past I also would've never shared my story, being too fearful of what people might think. However, according to The National

Alliance on Mental Illness, anxiety is the most prevalent mental health concern in the United States, affecting nearly 40 million adults (NAMI, 2017). Because of its prevalence, I don't feel so alone.

My goal for anyone that struggles with any form of anxiety is for them to find solace in the fact that they aren't alone. My goal is that more people feel comfortable voicing their concerns and be able to find a safe place to discuss them. There still is a large amount of stigma surrounding mental health, and I'm hoping it will significantly diminish by people opening up, deciding to share their stories, and advocating for acceptance. I want people to feel confident saying "I have anxiety. So what?" Please know, there is hope. Coming from someone who was convinced I would always be severely debilitated by anxiety, I'm telling you that doesn't have to be the case. Your mind is strong and beautiful and can open all kinds of doors. I'm happy to say I have finally found my way out of the revolving door and into the next chapter of my life. What will yours look like?

Exercise & Guiding Tips

The following is a short exercise and some simple guiding tips that helped me make changes in my life. Remember, this is what worked for me, and you need to ultimately find what works for you. If it's not this, that's okay, but hopefully it can spark some thoughts or lead you in the right direction. Also, remember wanting to make changes and being willing and implementing them are two different things. In the past I *wanted* to change, but I never did anything about it. My time came when it needed to, and so will yours. Have faith.

Exercise:

• Ask yourself:

1. What does my life look like right now (in terms of: your career, relationships, goals, etc.)?

2. Am I happy with my life?

3. What do I want my life to look like in 1 month...6 months...1 year?

> A. Does the way I'm living my life right now align with how I want my life to look like in 1 month...6 months...1 year?
>
> B. If not, why? What's holding me back?
>
> C. Am I willing to make changes in order to make them line up?

This exercise is merely meant as a starting point, and its objective isn't to overwhelm. This can be a lot to think about, so if you need to, look at one question at a time and come back to the others later.

· · ·

Guiding Tips:

1. Become aware and mindful of your thoughts. Try replacing any negative irrational thoughts with realistic or rational ones.

• Example:

Irrational thought: "Why hasn't he texted me back? He probably thought I was weird and won't ever talk to me again."

Rational thought: "Why hasn't he texted me back? He could be in class or in a meeting right now. He might text me later."

2. Try reframing the way you view a situation. For example, instead of viewing things as scary and intimidating, attempt to picture them as temporary challenges. This personally worked for me because I love a good challenge and that makes me more inclined to pursue it.

3. You may feel silly doing this at first, but try practicing positive self-affirmations. I always hated being told to do this, but guess who practices them now? This girl! It helps combat the negative self-talk that can chip away at your confidence.

• I can do it.
• I'm worth it.

- I have the power to create positive change for myself.

4. Find a healthy outlet to channel the anxiety, such as working out, journaling, joining a sports league, talking with a close friend, playing music, or painting. The anxiety will most likely fight against this, making it initially challenging to follow through and difficult to find motivation. Just stick with it and know it gets easier over time. It's well worth it.

5. One of the goals of social anxiety is to appear "normal" to society. This is accomplished by attempting to forestall any negative judgments people may have, consequently avoiding situations altogether or mitigating others' potential judgments by behaving in a way you believe will be accepted. It can be difficult opening up to people when the goal is to appear "normal," often leading to an isolated life. Have you ever held onto a secret that weighed you down, and you wanted to shout it off a rooftop? After sharing my experiences with some people, I felt similar to how I'd imagine that'd feel. The burden had been lifted. It's easier said than done, but my recommendation is to confide in someone you trust and to open up about any challenges you may be facing. The ability to currently be willing and able to share my thoughts with my family and friends has been invaluable and has helped immensely.

6. Fear is healthy and a part of life, so give yourself

permission to feel it. Avoiding it doesn't make it go away. I like to compare fear to traffic. You notice that one highway has heavy traffic due to construction, so you take another route, avoiding it altogether. However, despite avoiding it initially, you notice the same traffic jam is present on the return trip. The construction issue hasn't been resolved, so the traffic continues. Avoiding the issue does not make it go away. The construction needs to be completed, or the fear faced, in order for things to move more smoothly.

7. Attempt one challenge at a time, such as talking to someone new. It's okay to take baby steps, and it's more productive to take your time compared to pushing yourself to the point that you become overwhelmed. Take it one day at a time.

8. Celebrate victories and be kind to yourself with any difficulties along the way. All victories are amazing and deserve to be acknowledged. Let the mishaps go and give yourself a break.

As for me, I will continue to use these tips and to face the fear head on so that hopefully one day the anxiety will be able to come and go just like a gnat that I'm swatting away. I've gained incredible insight into myself during this process and have actually realized I don't need to get married or have kids in order to be happy. I'm having an incredible time simply experiencing life and am looking forward to what my 30s will bring.

"Worrying is like a rocking chair. It will give you something to do, but it won't get you anywhere." - proverb

National Alliance on Mental Illness (2017). Anxiety Disorders. Retrieved from https://www.nami.org/learn-more/mental-health-conditions/anxiety-disorders

ALLISON ROSE

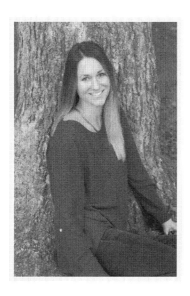

Allison Rose obtained her master's degree in clinical psychology and was given The Best Psychology Student Award in her undergraduate psychology class.

She is a Licensed Professional Clinical Counselor and Licensed Alcohol and Drug Counselor who possesses multiple years' experience as a clinician working with clients who struggle with severe and persistent mental illness, substance use, and complex medical concerns. She has worked in co-occurring treatment facilities and managed care.

Her expertise include substance use, anger management, working with offenders with increased criminogenic needs as well as other high-risk populations.

Allison enjoys engaging in volunteer activities that advocate for mental health. She co-coordinated fundraisers for NAMIWalk and is a former council member on the Advisory Council on Opioid Use Disorders in the African American Community.

If you have questions or want to know more, you can contact Allison on her LinkedIn page at:

https://www.linkedin.com/in/allison-rose-29a907ba/.

4

ASHLEIGH GUTHRIE

THE POWER OF SOUND

"To enter into the initiation of sound, vibration and mindfulness, is to take a giant step toward consciously knowing the soul."

Don G. Campbell, The Roar of Silence.

*M*y voyage of healing through sound began 3 years ago after the unexpected death of my mother in September 2016. My whole perception of life was altered with a single phone call.

I was on holiday in Africa at the time and was unable to return home for another week as we were in the middle of nowhere. Once back in London, through the turning of the key in the front door my rose-tinted glasses fell away and the veils of separation were lifted. I heard my soul calling me home.

The 3 year relationship that I was in at the time rapidly turned into a toxic, living nightmare, where I constantly felt like I was walking on eggshells, living with a Jekyll and Hyde character, when all I wanted, and needed, was to be held and told that I was safe. My experience of grief and the passing of my mother became entangled with my partner's narcissistic outbursts and emotional abuse, which resulted in me being diagnosed with Complex Post Traumatic Stress Disorder 12 months later.

Here in this chapter of 'The Power of Sound' I share with you an honest and open hearted adaptation of how sound, vibration, song and music has been such a huge part of my personal healing but how practically you can create your own sound healing experiences for yourself and loved ones. I have included exercises that can be used to amplify deeper connection, courage, freedom and joy in your life.

By combining various healing arts with science-based practices I now offer sound therapy and grief ceremonies both privately and in groups. From these offerings I have been a witness to sound and its ability to bring deep healing and transformation on a cellular level.

I found it particularly challenging when asked to write this chapter. Anyone who has suffered from CPTSD will likely be familiar with the sensations of trauma, fear, panic and dissociation that can arise when trying to recall memories from the past. It can feel like you are right back there, re-living the event. Therefore, as I write this, I am soothed by the sounds of nature, writing in the best way I know, from the heart.

During the first seven weeks after my mum's death, I remember trying to numb myself by watching Gossip Girl on repeat, listening to the theme song over and over again.....XOXO

It's amazing how we can use music to distract from our emotions and our thoughts. It can help us escape all the noise and constant chatter from the mind when we're not yet ready to feel and listen to what our hearts are aching to share because we are so immersed in the pain.

Fast forward 6 months to March 2017. I had reached a point where I had become so isolated, so alone and fear based that I was having panic attacks. On this particular day I was walking down the streets of Notting Hill when the panic set in. I clutched a wall unable to breathe and people walked past me like I didn't exist.

I felt totally unseen, completely alone and abandoned.

The result of this left me unable to leave the house the next day. I had reached the point of surrender, down on my knees, screaming internally, "I have nothing left to give".

And yet at the same time I had this deep inner question burning within my heart, "What am I here for? What's my purpose?".

I was finally ready to listen.

I sat for over four hours in silence and prayed for the first time in my life, calling to something greater than myself, over and over again.

"What am I here for? What's my purpose?"

It was like something out of one of my favourite films - Eat, Pray, Love.

I had done very little meditation and never picked up a spiritual book at that point.

Eventually from the silence the answer came - "Go back to working with the senses, discover how to release emotions from the body".

Although I'd been a masseuse for over 10 years, at that point mind-body connection was a completely new concept to me.

I realised at that moment that something had to change, and that something was me. There was no knight in shining armour coming to save me. I had been placing my happiness on the shoulders of another which was an unrealistic expectation and it was then that I realised that "only I am responsible for my happiness, therefore I'm not responsible for anyone else's happiness."

And so, I CHOSE the leap of faith and dived into the depth of the unknown. I CHOSE to shift my focus from fear to curiosity towards the mysteries of spirituality, sound healing, mind-set and shamanic ceremony.

My mum's death catapulted me onto this vision quest of searching of the soul, remembering that it calls one back to wholeness. I knew that one day when I was ready, I would help others find joy on the other side of suffering. But first I had to go on my own healer's journey, and it was clear that this had to be through the power of sound.

As I began working with spiritual life coach, Michelle Zelli, I became aware of the fears that had been triggering the panic attacks, predominantly the fear of abandonment. I felt supported and started to re-educate myself on how to let go of the stories I was telling myself that were keeping me trapped in fear.

By becoming acutely aware of my internal "stories", implementing daily rituals and looking out for mini miracles during my day, I found enough courage to leave the toxic relationship and I bought a ticket to Bali.

My favourite method to feel into and release fear is to take a "Sensory Soul Shower."

I invite you to either visualise or after reading this, actually go take a shower.

Taking a few deep breaths into your heart, begin by massaging your finest shower oils/body wash into your skin and immerse yourself under this cleansing shower. Bring your attention to the sound of the water falling from above, allowing yourself to be held within this safe space. Releasing all tension, quieting the mind, becoming aware of your body and the aromas within this sacred shower.

When you're ready call in your soul and ask "What's the fear? What am I afraid to let go of? Why am I resisting?".

This is a conversation between you and your soul, breathing in patience with your inhale, releasing judgment with your exhale.

Listen with compassion to the answers that are revealed. Take however long feels right for you to receive.

Then ask yourself, "Is this true?".

When you're ready, take a deep breath and begin to visualise the water cascading over you as a beautiful, cleansing white light, washing away any fear, doubt, judgment, resentment, anger or pain from every single cell within your magnificent body, purifying the mind and ego which has been trying so hard to protect you. Connect into your heart, take a deep breath and visualise or sense luminous liquid gold being poured deep within your heart. Breathe in unconditional love.

You are safe

You are enough

You are love

Listen to your heart, the wisdom will follow.

I feel immense gratitude for everything I have experienced over the last few years, both the painful and the beautiful. I have given myself time and space to heal, and in return I have rediscovered my passion for travel and a hunger for knowledge.

This has guided me around the globe in search of how to integrate the mystical, eastern philosophies and healing arts as I'm aware that not everyone has access to these opportunities. It brings me great joy to share these teachings and integrate them into the western world by creating sensory soul experiences that stir the soul to find deeper connection, peace of mind and freedom from suffering.

I've learnt that suffering can cease but it doesn't necessarily mean pain will stop. Every once in a while, the Universe will throw you a test to see if you are listening; "Are you committed?". Sometimes the lessons are still painful, but there's a difference between pain and suffering. I believe suffering is a choice. You can choose to let go of the attachment and surrender fears. It's like the Universe is saying..."Show me your new vibration and I will show you my miracles".

I think that's when you come into exploring your own mental health by playfully exploring and learning how to incorporate more mindful thinking based practices, grounding tools that you can draw upon when you're being triggered so that you feel safe to be in your body, creating daily rituals that inspire you every day, to bring about more self-acceptance, forgiveness, compassion and self-discovery that assists you in this lifelong journey of rebirth.

After Bali I had a deep intuitive soul calling that I was to go to Nepal and learn how to play the Tibetan Singing Bowls, bring them home and combine them with massage and meditation. I found myself living at a monastery for over a month with monks and nuns studying Buddhist psychology, meditation and mantras. My soul suddenly felt alive!

During this time, I was fortunate enough to find Tibetan Shamans who taught me how to play the Tibetan Singing Bowls. They passed on their grandfathers' teachings and showed me how the vibrations from the bowls can shift blockages on both an energetic and physical level. These teachings were a combination of highly intuitive skills passed down through generations, combined with energy and science-based theory.

When the external vibration comes into your body from the singing bowls, it allows you to become fully present from within, allowing you to connect with your own unique vibration. It's like nothing else exists in that moment. It evokes a childlike curiosity and playfulness. Sound healing gives you space to just be. It allows you to notice what is happening internally from a place of peace as you feel into the vibration and allow the sounds to create waves of calmness.

I have found that sound allows you to explore who you are as a person, what feels good and nurturing, as well as what feels uncomfortable and overwhelming. There will be sounds that you don't like, but it's all about raising awareness to who you are. It brings an opportunity to explore your own emotional range and vitality of what is going on internally.

Language is built on sound, our identity is built on sound; our names hold great power, and so the idea is that we are each a unique being, expressing our personal song into the Universe as we connect into our essence, our individual sound, vibration and frequency.

The vibration from the Tibetan Singing Bowls loosens density within the body. Fellow sound healer and astrologer Daniel Alzamora explains; "Think of a jack-hammer, as it beats into the surface it vibrates free attachments. Vibration is a carrier wave for intention. It can either strengthen bonds, or it can dissolve them.

This is how it can help you either loosen bonds of things that you wish to liberate and let go of, or it can strengthen the bonds of unity and togetherness. I believe that sound healing allows you to become conscious of your inner world and acts as a carrier to project it out into the universe."

As you start to raise your own vibration you may find that your language starts to change, your taste in music alters, people and material things that were once important to you may begin to fall away. As you become more aware of your internal world, start to notice how your external environment starts to align to your higher frequency.

Sound = Vibration

Vibration = Light

Frequency = Intention

Low vibration emotions - Shame, guilt, fear anger

High vibration emotions - Love, peace, joy, gratitude

"The mind and the body are connected".

I was recently introduced to the concept of psychoacoustics, a study showing how sounds affect the immune function, a scientific exploration of the mind body connection. This fascinates me because the women from my mother's lineage have a history of autoimmune disease. My grandmother had Multiple Sclerosis and my mother was diagnosed the year I was born which means that on a cellular level there was a high probability that MS could have been passed down to me.

In my experience I have found that by combining psychological practices such as hypnotherapy (meditation with intention) with sound and vibrational healing we can not only heal our own childhood wounds at a cellular level, but with an intent we can also create frequencies that release molecular imbalances within our family lineage.

Some of these emotional releases can be very painful so we usually tend to repress them deep within, where we can't feel them again. No matter how intense and painful a release might be, we ultimately feel much better afterwards. The more we clear ourselves from accumulated lower frequency emotions, the higher our frequency will rise and the happier and healthier we'll become on a cellular level.

In order to raise our own vibration to match that of higher emotional frequencies, so that we may embody more love and joy, we must first become aware of our language, the company we keep and our environments.

I invite you in this moment to reflect on situations when you hear certain music and sounds during your daily life or perhaps feel into your current environment if you are out in public. Just take a moment to pause and ponder....

Perhaps you are within a restaurant, on a bus, the tube or maybe you are driving whilst listening to the radio.

Do you make judgments about whether you like the sounds or not?

Can you recall a time when you have overheard parents having a conversation with their children, have you ever made judgments on the language they use?

We all have an inner voice that tells us whether we're 'good' or 'bad', what's 'naughty' or 'nice' based upon our belief systems that have been dictated by our upbringing and the status quo.

I like to think of them as the little devil and angel you see in the Tom and Jerry cartoons.

The inner critic - the fear based ego that passes judgments throughout the day, repeating stories and false beliefs from childhood trauma and subsequent life experiences that keep you feeling unworthy of love, blaming others for your unhappiness which as a result keep you trapped in the cycle of suffering as 'the victim.'

The higher self - the highest vibrational version of you who speaks the truth of who and what you really are, the soul. It is your connection to the unconscious. It is you at the purest level.

Allow yourself to take a moment of stillness, close your eyes, turn your focus inwards and take a few deep breaths. Relax into your body.

Take your time and allow yourself to become
of your thoughts, just listen.

What is your inner critic telling you at this
time?

Connect into your heart by taking a few breaths and ask
yourself, is it true?

What false, low vibration judgements are you ready to
let go of?

Now, take a cleansing breath in for four seconds, hold for
four and release anything that no longer serves you
exhaling with the sound of AAAAAHHHHHH!!! Try
this for seven breaths.

As you are sounding this tone, feel the sound projecting
unconditional love from the centre of your chest. Feel
yourself being at peace.

Allow yourself to rest in silence for a few moments to
perceive any changes that may have occurred from
within your being.

Now, from this place of silence, using your imagination
start to call in the intention to connect with your higher
self, by visualising a beautiful healing white light,
rimmed with fluorescent violet, feel or sense it cleansing
and purifying every single cell within your mind and
body.

Ask your higher self, what is my heart yearning for?

.llow yourself to soften and listen deeper.....

The higher self whispering its pearls of wisdom to soothe your soul.

Let the fears and doubts dissolve within the abundance and frequency of compassion that are spoken with these words now.

You are enough and you are wanted.

You are a child of light and divinity.

You are worthy of love because you are love.

My beautiful blazing angel.

Energy follows thought, sound healing can evoke moments of peace that help the inner critic to fall away which has a huge impact on re-training your thought patterns, create space to connect in and listen to your higher self for guidance when calling in your intentions for manifesting your deepest hearts desires.

The Tibetan Shamans explained how the frequencies from the bowls match the same brain wave frequencies (intentions) that we use when we go into deep states of meditation, allowing the mind and body to fall into deeper states of balance, relaxation, well-being and wholeness. This is known as brainwave entrainment.

Entrainment synchronises our fluctuating brainwaves by providing a stable frequency which the brainwave can attune to. By using vibration and frequency we can entrain our brainwaves and it then becomes possible to relax our normal beta state (normal waking consciousness) to alpha (relaxed consciousness), it is here we can reach theta (meditative state) and delta (sleep; where internal healing can occur).

We are constantly being influenced and therefore fine tuning the rhythms of our body and consciousness through the vibrations we encounter within our environments. Our bodies have many different rhythms and sound effects, these are through our voice, breathing, heart rate and digestion.

By becoming aware and contemplating our emotions, our body and our thought pattern, whilst experiencing sound and vibration, we can retrain our nervous system and brain waves to enhance our personal lives through reducing stress and anxiety and heightening our consciousness through the senses.

Our voice holds great power.

Everything in the Universe is pulsating and vibrating – nothing is really standing still!

Vibrations and rhythms can have a physical effect on the body by slowing down the nervous system and entraining the brain waves similar to the singing bowl meditation. When the mind is relaxed, your blood pressure decreases and ultimately the health of your heart improves.

When you sing, musical vibration moves through you, altering your physical and emotional state. Singing is innate, ancient and within all of us. I have found it to be one of the most uplifting therapeutic things we can do. You do not have to be an amazing singer to feel the benefits, and with practice your state of flow increases.

During my time in Guatemala I experienced something called Kirtan. I have never seen so many people coming together from a place of pureness and wholeheartedness. I felt like a small child mesmerised by the love being chanted through the words of devotional singing.

According to Kirtan artist and bhakti yoga educator David Newman, Kirtan means "to praise that which is exalted"— aka, the divine. The word "Kirtan" also stems from a Sanskrit root that means "to cut through," he says, so Kirtan is also "a practice for cutting through the idea of separation, for connecting to our hearts and connecting to the moment through sound."

Singing in groups triggers the communal release of serotonin and oxytocin, the bonding hormone, and even synchronises our heart beats which can aid towards relieving anxiety and stress. Singing together not only brings happiness, but deeply connects people on a soul level. It helps people with depression and reduces feelings of loneliness, leaving people feeling relaxed, joyful and free.

According to one study in America, "Sixty-two women and men with an average age of 50 reported significantly less tension, anger, fatigue, and depressed mood after experiencing sound meditation sessions".

My time in Peru lead me on a magical voyage of sound and nature. The amazon was a beautiful reminder of how all living creatures are constantly singing their unique soul song, reminding us to be grateful that we are alive. The earth and the skies were filled with life; sound in motion. During the shamanic ceremonies, healing songs known as Icaros would be sung, guided by the maestro shaman.

They would cleanse us with their voices, calling in their ancestors for protection, guiding us like singing shepherds as we journeyed into the depths of the subconscious realms. These sacred songs are used to give thanks to Pachamama, Mother Earth for her nurturing medicines.

There are different kinds and each one has their own unique power and purpose, the vibrations of these medicine songs can rearrange the frequency (intention) of your energy systems, conjuring harmonic wholeness.

I believe that everybody can sing so let the soul songs flow out wherever you are.

When asked what song I wanted to play at my mother's funeral for her final send off, I had just watched the film "Wild" with Reece Weatherspoon. It shares the story of her soul pilgrimage after the death of her mother and the song that was played throughout the film was El Condor Pasa (If I could) by Simon and Garfunkel.

I have fond childhood memories of my mum and Aunty Alison singing Simon and Garfunkel songs together in the car and so I found myself listening with different ears as there was now a deeper meaning taking place within my heart's ears.

The Multiple Sclerosis had taken effect on my mother's ability to walk for as long as I could remember, so when I heard the lyrics "I'd rather feel the earth beneath my feet. Yes, I would, if I only could, I surely would." I knew this was the song to choose.

As I started to fine tune my awareness to the language within songs, I noticed how it had a profound effect on how I was coping with my own mental health, anxiety and grief. It began to feel like my mum could communicate to me through the lyrics of song, soothing the young girl inside, my inner child, who was yet to connect to the grief and realisation that her mum was no longer here on earth.

Music became my soul's medicine. I noticed I was being drawn to songs that allowed me to open my heart, this allowed me to trust that it was safe to express my love to another through the magic of music as I had struggled to share what I was feeling verbally.

I met a beautiful soul sister who quickly became my muse. We started to exchange daily voice notes, sharing our spiritual musings and how we were feeling, I found this to be a liberating practice of open, honest and non-judgmental communication.

My experience with talking therapy was extremely stressful. I struggled to put into words how I was feeling, I felt like I was repeating the same story, bringing back feelings of isolation and entrapment. These soul musings helped me to become aware of when I was speaking from my inner critic or from my higher self and I began to feel less alone, I felt seen, heard and loved from a place of uncondition.

I share this technique to evoke a time of reflection to think about whom might there be in your life that you would consider a muse for your souls' expression? Someone to share your thoughts and feelings with, with no fear of judgment?

I began to create playlists with titles of intent that aligned with the emotions that were arising for us both, I would choose songs that spoke to the pain and fear, yet at the same time offering hope and liberation. I rediscovered some of the world's greatest love songs and offered them wholeheartedly, to my soul muse, observing what she needed to hear in order to take the leap of faith.

"You are safe"

"You are wanted"

"You are loved"

"You are brave"

"You are courageous"

"You are strength"

"You are beautiful"

It was through the graceful act of giving and receiving that formed a beautiful soul-based union, giving space for separation and loneliness to fall away.

Using your soul muse as your inspiration, send them a voice note and ask them how they are feeling today. If anything, you will be doing an act of kindness by brightening up your friend's day showing them that someone cares.

Begin by exploring your choice of music platform as you start to structure your unique sound medicine. All of my playlists are public on Spotify.

I invite you to listen with a clearer perspective, with fresh ears. Go deeper within the lyrics, using this exercise to have a tangible conversation with the soul or perhaps a loved one who is no longer of this world, connecting through the sensations of sound medicine.

Now that you have your playlist you can invite in the soul to dance with you.

Dance is another way in which we can give ourselves permission to let the inner critic and ego mind to fall away, giving freedom of expression to the higher self, like the birthing a beautiful butterfly, as it expands its wings in poetic flight. A canvas for ecstatic liberation.

When dancing alone, call in the healing light of your higher self, visualise your soul reflecting back at you, giving spirit human form, freedom to speak the language of love and emotion through your beautiful body of sound, frequency and vibration.

Movement in motion can connect us as one heart.

Beat by beat.

I invite you to play your playlist on shuffle and become aware of how your body wants to move.

Notice any areas of tension, restriction.

Where in your body do you feel fluid and free?

Notice any sensations that may be stirred from as you dance, uniting mind, body and soul.

Allow your body to become attuned to the melodic rhythm, feel the beat stirring from within, pulsating subliminal sensations that quiver your unlimited state of being into artistic self-expression through dance, music, pleasure, joy.

And then..........come to a place of stillness and just rest.

There is great power in silence; it is from this space of stillness that deep healing takes place.

When we sing the language of love and breathe together as one, we are raising the vibration to heal our planet. Mother Earth at this time needs us to become aware of our own healing frequencies (intentions) and invites us to step forward, awaken and unite.

It is my deepest heart's desire that this book brings enlightenment to those who are curious enough to step into their light and join together as a conscious community of wellbeing warriors.

ASHLEIGH GUTHRIE

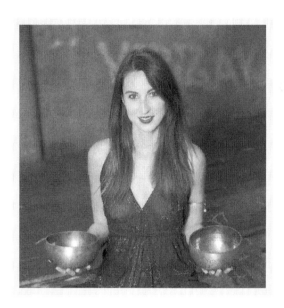

Ashleigh Guthrie is a sound healer, grief ceremonialist and spiritual coach known for her deep dive, hypnotic healing experiences.

At the age of 24, she was the founder of Manchester's number one day spa and finalist for the regions Young Entrepreneur Award within her first year of trading.

With over a decade in the health and wellness industry, Ashleigh brings to life unique sensory immersions that stir the soul through the senses. Her medicine bag includes a wide range of techniques including sound healing with Tibetan Singing Bowls, hypnosis, breath work and intuitive massage. Her offerings can assist with grief, trauma, womb and sexual healing allowing more space for personal growth and self-acceptance.

Ashleigh, follows her passion for travelling and thirst for knowledge on mysticism, mindset and mind-body connection.

This has led her to work on retreats across the globe, exploring massage techniques in the temple where Buddha was massaged, qualifying as a sound therapist from Tibetan Shamans as well as learning Meditation techniques in Nepal whilst living with Monks and Nuns.

She works around the UK and overseas on a one-to-one basis, and with groups creating ceremonies for both men and women to amplify connection, accelerate transformation, empowering people to live radiantly with more courage, freedom and joy.

Website

www.ashleighguthrie.com

Instagram

@thesensorysoul

Facebook

Ashleigh Guthrie - Sensory Soul Experiences

facebook.com/ashleigh.guthrie

instagram.com/ashleighguthrie

5

CARLSTON MEDFORD

BECOMING THE PERSON I LOVE

"You are who you choose to be"

Ted Hughes

*I*t is said that your beliefs shape who you are, and that between the ages of 2 years and 4 years is when you start to form your beliefs. Whether true or not, I believed once you become an adult, you are free to change, add or get rid of any belief you deemed fit, providing you have identified the belief you want to change and you have a strong enough reason for that change.

Growing up for me was hard and it felt lonely. I did not feel as though my parents loved me and my conclusion was that I was not deserving of love. The chapter to follow will explain how I managed to change my point of view and become the person I am today, the person that I love.

Self-Criticism: We learn by analysing everything that happens to us, in order to gauge every experience. For example, if we lift an object, we can determine if it is heavy or light depending on our capacity to exert the muscular strength needed to lift said object. Based on what we decide, we may be able to lift it on our own, may need assistance or choose not to lift it altogether.

Another option may be to train our muscles over a period of time and attempt to lift the object once we have increased our strength. Self-criticism is quite similar to this concept. We compare ourselves to others and sometimes we are of the opinion we are not good enough in comparison.

Some people choose to work at improving who they are all on their own, some ask for help, while others do nothing about it and continue to see themselves as less than worthy.

I once saw myself as less than in comparison to others. I was too short, too skinny, too ugly, no one liked me, everything happens to me and most of all I did not feel love from my parents.

Limiting Beliefs: As mentioned just ahead of this paragraph, all the self-criticism I had about myself was created within my unconsciousness and is what I called my limiting beliefs. For example, being considered short meant being picked on by taller people. Being skinny meant I was physically weak.

Being ugly, well you get the point. This was how I saw myself and despite being told by friends and some family that it was not the case, it did not change the way I felt towards myself. I would say to myself that they are just trying to make me feel better, but I know the truth and the feeling of nothing would not go away.

Every day I saw this, I heard this in my head, and I felt this in my soul, and no one could have changed my point of view. These ideas about myself influenced my behaviour as well. For example, I got into a fight once at school just because a boy, who was older and bigger than I was, looked at me longer than I thought he should have.

In my mind he was sizing me up and preparing to attack, so my reaction to my perception was to attack first. Well I got the first strike but did not win the battle. Despite my short comings (laughing at myself), I continued with this behaviour for some time until I realised fighting was not my best plan of action, especially when it appeared that I kept finding bigger opponents than myself.

I also never had the courage to speak to girls in my teenage years, as I feared they would say no to liking a short skinny boy who always seems to be angry at the slightest thing. I was even told once by my mother, I would end up in prison due to my temper. You see, what you **Experience** times what you **Believe** equals your **Behaviour**.

The funny thing about your beliefs are that whatever you think, will affect how you see the world around you, and everything you see will confirm what you think. For example, I thought being small meant being an easy target, which lead to my action of fighting, which lead to my result of losing (not all the time), which lead to my belief of being an easy target. Below is a diagram that best explain this cycle of behaviour.

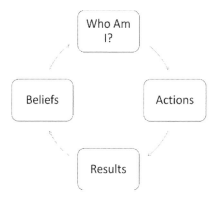

The decision: One of my good qualities, at least what I consider a good quality, is my level of stubbornness. I was determined not to prove my mother correct by ending up in jail. I was always respectful to everyone I thought deserved it but knew that if I did not manage my anger issues that I might hear my mum say, "Yup I was right about you" and that was never going to happen in my reality.

On my 16th birthday I stood in front of the bathroom mirror and said to myself, "you are a man now and you must work at being someone you love", as being who I was for the last 16 years would not do.

The thought of spending another 16 years being myself, as I was then, was too sad to think of. I knew who I did not want to be any more but who to become was the big question.

Seeing that I saw myself as less than, and that I told myself I was not good enough I often felt less than adequate, so I decided that I would have to learn how to see myself better than I did, say better things to myself and feel good about myself and the only way I knew, at the time, was to pay attention to people around me and identify those with the qualities I was looking for.

Modelling: The first person I decided to pay attention to was my Sunday school teacher, Mr Williams who always dressed well, always had a smile on his face and I got along with him pretty well. I decided that whenever I was going anywhere that I would always dress smart and walk with a smile on my face.

This was easier said than done as I did not have a lot of clothes to choose from and changing my habit of trying to look tough as a means to self-defence took some time and effort but eventually I began to come around. After a while I noticed that I didn't feel as angry as I usually did and that more and more people, who I did not know, would pass me and smile back at me. This was the beginning of me building my confidence and self-worth.

Associations: Throughout my school years I had developed a network of good friends of which I am still close too at present. I was told by my mum, in my younger years, that following friends will get me into trouble. I had decided then to be careful when choosing my friends as I could not allow my mum to be right about me, (as I said, stubborn).

Me and my friends studied together, played together, stole mangoes together, as kids would do, but generally looked after each other. Some of us even went to college together and because of the great friendship we had built throughout school, the support needed for college studies was there to tap into.

It has been mentioned by millionaires that the two most important things that will influence a person are the books they read and the people they associate with. In my life I can say that I have found this to be true. I have children of my own now and I have sat down with them and explained that a good friend is anyone who adds value to their lives in a positive way, such as giving good advice which is based on evidence.

A good friend will let you know you are wrong, even if

you do not want to admit it to yourself. Always put a smile on your face even when they are not present and make you feel like a person of worth. They will never encourage you to do something that you know to be wrong.

This is the judging ruler I use when selecting a friend and I hope whoever is reading this chapter finds this to be helpful as well. You can go online these days to find positive motivational books to read, you can even listen to them if you do not like reading so there is no excuse any more for not educating yourself in the ways to becoming a happy person.

Focus: I hope by now you are realising that in order for you or anyone to make positive changes in your life you have got to begin with the idea that change can occur, and most importantly it can occur within you. If you do not come to this realisation yourself, nothing I am saying here will make a difference. All I can say is, if I could manage to change my unwanted behaviour, I am positive you are more than capable of doing the same, that is if you really want to.

I want you to try an experiment. I want you to stand in the centre of a room that you are not familiar with and as you stand in the centre of the room with this book in your hand, I want you to slowly look around the room and moving in any direction, I want you to observe everything that is red.

Once you have done that, I want you to stand still and focus your eyes back onto this book. Follow the dots you are about to see and then answer the question at the end of the dots...

without looking up and around the room what was the colour of the wall behind you ?

If you got it right without looking congratulations, if you did not then that is ok, I did not get it right the first time either.

Most people do not see anything else than what they focus on. This happens because our mind deals with information in three (3) ways: By deleting, generalising and distorting the information we are receiving. By focusing on the red items only, our mind deleted all other information it deemed unnecessary. If you understand this process, then you can understand the point I am trying to make.

If you focus on being an unhappy person you will see all the information and evidence around you to support the fact that you are an unhappy person. Even saying things to yourself such as I do not want to be unhappy can still cause you to be unhappy, as your unconscious mind will only hear unhappy and not the phrase "I do not want".

What I recommend to everyone is that when you get up in the morning, before even getting out of bed, list ten (10) things you are grateful for having in your life. Examples are I am grateful my heart is beating, I am grateful I am breathing, I am grateful I still have my mobility, you get the idea now.

What this does is train your unconscious mind on focusing on things to be happy about and not the reverse. Once I learnt to be grateful for what I had and not focus on what I do not have, I started to see better ways to achieve my personal goals and happiness.

Respect: "A feeling of deep admiration for someone or something elicited by their abilities, qualities or achievements, also described as a regard for the feelings, wishes or rights of others", as described by the Oxford dictionary. My simple way of explaining respect is to treat yourself and others the best way you can. I also advocate accepting nothing less than respect from others as well.

Once I started to pay attention to my behaviour, my thoughts, my actions and realised that I was becoming someone who I felt great about and who others felt great about too, I started to see myself in a different way. I noticed the internal voice in my head was a happier voice and was more patient with me.

I also noticed when I looked into the mirror, I smiled lots more to myself and had a warm feeling inside my body which accompanied these feelings. I realised that myself respect was growing and that I loved it. What I also noticed is that when my respect for myself increased the way people treated me also changed, not to say they treated me badly in the first place, but my opinions seemed to be considered more than before.

I realised that people's opinions did not have to be the same as mine and that we can still have a civil conversation without arguments. If only I had learnt this years earlier, I could have saved myself loads of grief but as I have come to learn, every experience in life can teach you a lesson only if you are open to the idea of learning and you pay attention.

Health and Fitness: Let me start by saying I am not a health and fitness instructor nor am I a dietician. What I can say is when I paid attention to what I ate and exercised more, I felt physically better in myself, began to look physically better and had loads of energy. I do believe that when we focus on this aspect of our life, not only does your physical fitness improve, your mental health also improves.

Something that I will ask everyone who is reading this chapter to do, is to go and find professional practitioners in health such as Doctors or fitness instructors, to verify what I am saying. If you can gather the correct information from qualified and professional people, then you can make a better assessment of what I am saying with the hope of taking action.

My journey started with me writing down what I ate, how much I ate, what time I ate and how active my day was. I will be honest I did not keep this up for long (the writing I meant), I eventually realised that I could eat whatever I liked just as long as I remained active and did not eat in excess, I was good.

Now that was my personal experience, yours may be different as no two human beings are exactly the same, but I am sure that it will be of worth to you to find out what is the best eating program for your body to operate at its best, and what impact it can have on your mental state.

Conclusion: Now I hope that after all you have read you have come to understand all the things that I have considered in the remaking of myself. I started in my teens and I am still practising everything that I mentioned. I would admit I am not as physically active as I used to be and a bit rounder than I care to admit, but generally I am the same person that I worked so hard at creating. I can look in the mirror and say, "I love you" to myself and really mean it.

I would say that there are two struggles I experienced. The first was to become the person I wanted to be; the next struggle is to maintain the person I have become. Once you have made the necessary changes to your thinking that will give you the results you are looking for, you may notice that the people around you may look different. I do not mean physically; I mean in their behaviour. It is so funny that by changing the way you look at situations, you can see something totally different.

Realise that because you are willing to change not everyone you associate with will do the same, if you come across a situation where the people around you seem to be pulling you back to where you were at first, it is just because they do not know any better and you should not hold it against them but at the same time, I would advise you keep focused on your end goal and let no one stop you from your task of becoming the person you want to be.

G.R.O.W model: This is a process that can help you to determine what changes to consider in order to become the person you want to be.

Goal : Who do you want to be? What do you want to change/improve? How important would it be to you for change to happen? When would you like this change to happen? Why do you want this change?

My "Why" was probably the driving force behind every action I have mentioned in this chapter. For me living my life for another 16 years and feeling the same way I did at the time, was not how I wanted my life to be. Why? Because I absolutely hated feeling a lack of love from my parents, but most of all from myself. I knew that I could feel different as there were times that I did, but what I wanted was to feel good about myself all the time. I just had to work out the How.

Reality: In order to get to where you want to go you

need to know where you are. Ask yourself questions like What is going on in your life now? When does this happen? What causes it? When did it happen? How does it affect you? (on a scale of 1-10, 1 being the least affected 10 being the most affected). By understanding the things that are affecting you, you are understanding what needs to be worked on.

An exercise which is helpful but can also be hard to do, because it asks you to be totally honest with yourself, is to get an A4 size sheet of paper and fold it vertically with the line running from top to bottom, through the centre of the sheet. On one half I want you to write all the things you like about yourself, and then on the other half, I want you to write all the things you do not like about yourself. Make this list as thorough as possible and do not be afraid to put everything on, even if it hurts. Remember this is your list and no one else has to see it.

Options: At this stage these are the questions to start asking yourself. What can be done to get better results? What might someone else do in the same situation? How have you overcome similar situations in the past? What is needed for you to achieve your desired outcome? Where can you get help and from who? How can you do it?

By asking yourself questions you are engaging your unconscious mind to start searching for answers. Our mind is fantastic at problem solving only if we allow it to. Next, what I want you to do is to look at your sheet of paper where you wrote down all the things that you did not like about yourself and ask yourself, for each dislike, what can I do to either make this better or get rid of it all together. Use options to figure out how you can deal with all your dislikes in a very affective way.

Way Forward: Question to ask yourself. What are your next steps? When will you start? Who else do you need to involve? How confident are you in gaining your desired results? How will this fit in with your present situation? Who will you become?

Remember a sat nav cannot get you to your destination unless it has a point of origin where it begins from and a point of final destination. Sometimes you will encounter obstacles in the road but as we know, a sat nav is design to re-calculate, still allowing you to reach your destination. This is the same principle when working on improving yourself. It may not always go to plan, but once you re-calculate your direction, you will eventually get there.

I hope reading this chapter has really help you to see that whatever you are going through in life, it is only a perception of your reality and that you can change your perception, thus changing your reality. I hope you have come to the realisation that you are who you choose to be and that you can choose to be better than you presently are, but only if you choose too. By choosing to be better, you are giving yourself permission to start repairing what was damaged or what was wrong with you.

You are not in competition with anyone else only with the you of yesterday, for today you are a little bit better and tomorrow you will be even better than today. Remember to start your day with at least 10 things to be grateful for, look into the mirror and say to your reflection, "You are worthy of your own love". Say it with a smile on your face and make sure to be standing up right with your shoulders back. The reason I am saying this to you is that there is a direct connection between your emotional state and your physiology (the way you position your body).

To check this theory out, I want you to think of a moment you felt really sad about an event and as you picture that event, I want you to notice how your shoulders are positioned. I also want you to notice where your eyes are looking and how you are feeling inside. Try to smile and see if it feels natural. I hope you get the point that when you are feeling down or hurt about an event, your physical state matches your emotional state.

Shake your hands and head as if you were dancing. This is to break the state you just put yourself through then I want you to focus on an event where you felt really happy and even had a great time. Pay attention now to how your shoulders are different, notice where your eyes are looking as well as if you are smiling. Once you notice these changes ask yourself what has changed in order to get these different responses and I am sure you will deduce the connection between what we think and how we feel.

With this knowledge in mind you now have a tool that you can use to change your unhappy state at any time you care too. All the things I have mentioned in this chapter I have found to be simple to understand but not always easy to do.

The real challenge is to form them into a habit, and to do them. I will say once you make the conscious decision to work on becoming a better you, the next step can be to pick a few of my suggestions and practice them for the next (90) days. In your own time keep adding to your progress and eventually you will become the person you love.

As I sit here writing this book recalling my own experiences, I am feeling a warm sensation inside of myself which is coming from the result of my personal growth throughout the years. I hope that you, the reader of this chapter, can also look forward to the day you feel this sense of personal achievement and self-love.

Know that how you felt up to this point does not have to continue into your future, defining who you are. The phrase "You are not your behaviour" simply means your behaviour does not dictate who you are, only you can dictate that and only you can change your behaviour.

To you the person reading this chapter, my respect and admiration to you for investing time and knowledge into your personal growth. You are already on your way to becoming the person that you love, simply by adding this information to your life skills. Not only will I encourage you to put these skills to the test, I will ask you to pass on these suggestions to anyone you think may benefit from what you yourself have benefited from as well.

With all that said, do have a wonderful day.

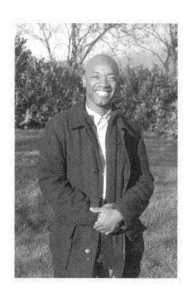

Carlston Medford was born and raised on the Island of Barbados. He grew up amongst family members who experienced mental health issues.

The issues varied from **Schizophrenia** to depression and bipolar disorder. He himself has experienced periods of depression and low self-esteem but through sheer determination and researching self-help methods he was able to change his pattern of thinking which affected his behaviour in a way that gave him his desired outcome.

Due to his familiarity with engaging those affected by mental health issues, he found that he had the ability to get others to open up to him and speak about their issues in a calm and safe manner.

For many years he wanted to study Psychology but fearing that he did not have what it took to study he refused to move forward within this field. It was only in 2018, after being told by many, if not all of his daily delivery customers, that he should be a counsellor because they found it easy to talk to him about their personal issues and how his suggestions seem to be easy to understand and implement. He decided to find a program that suited his study style and also something that seemed effective in producing positive results in those experiencing mental health issue.

He was introduced to NLP(Neuro Linguistic Programming) by a friend and after researching its applications as an alternative way in dealing with mental health, he then studied and became a practitioner of NLP which was ANLP accredited then went on to become a Master practitioner of NLP.

Since his qualifications, he has worked with clients on a 1 to 1 basis. His clients fall into the categories of depression, anxiety, family relations and even phobias. His style of coaching is a combination of NLP and good old fashioned empathy which allows him to connect with the client and offer possible tools to assist the client in reaching their desired outcome.

At present, Carlston is working on several training courses to assist those who are struggling to find within themselves harmony and self-love, both in their daily lives as well as their professional lives. Keep following his progress, contact him or share his details with anyone you think may be in need of his services.

He can be contacted through his website:

www.thehappyguy.co.uk ,

email address : info@thehappyguy.co.uk.

contact number +447397960677.

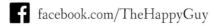 facebook.com/TheHappyGuy

6

CATE MCMURRAY

IDENTITY IS YOUR OWN BRAND OF MAGICK

*D*o you know who you are? As in, *really* know who you are? From the top of your head right down to your toes? Inside and out?

I didn't. It wasn't until I finally uncovered, and showed up, as the person I really am, that I understood how much not knowing or being "me" had impacted my life, and a lot of the choices I made up to that point.

From an early age I felt different to everyone else. Things that other children seemed to enjoy or find easy, I just didn't. My mum always said I was an easy child, and yet others that looked after me would tell her the opposite. She thought I was perfect (as most mothers do their children), but even she knew I was "different".

She would take me to see the Doctor and tell him that "something" wasn't right, and she would always get told that I was fine and to stop worrying, which of course she never did.

At the age of five I started seeing and hearing dead people. It sounds harsh, but that's exactly what it was for me at that point. I was still tiny but people that I knew weren't "real", would whisper things in my ear or show themselves to me when I was alone. It was scary and confusing and as I grew older, I convinced myself that there was something wrong with me so I kept it to myself.

Making friends wasn't my strong point, although I'm sure that some of the people I went to school with would say it didn't seem that way. Maintaining friendships felt even harder. I always felt like I was on the periphery looking into relationships that other people could have, but that I would never quite manage. I was bullied a lot by children my own age and a couple who were older, and over the years I started to believe some of the things they said about me, because that's the way it works, right?

I grew up in an amazing place, one that I look back at in wonder. My parents ran a snooker club and the building was one of stature. We occupied the warren-like ground floor with its huge rooms, flagstone floors and fairy-tale sweeping staircase with matching mahogany handrail that my sisters and I would slide all the way down, when Mum wasn't looking.

The Minton tiled hallway always captivated me. It's

ridiculously high ceiling and enormous width made it incredibly echoey, and every time I needed a new pair of shoes, I hoped that they would "clip-clop" so that I could hear that sound whenever I walked through it. Of course, my shoes never made any noise; the rubber soles of a small schoolgirl's shoes weren't conducive to any kind of clip-clopping at all, but I always hoped.

School didn't become any easier as time went on, in fact it felt more isolating than ever, and I dreaded every single day of it.

The people I could hear, that no one else could, got louder, and along with their ever-increasing noise came visions in the form of dreams - always bad ones. I would wake up crying and scared, with a feeling of dread filling my body and whilst my mum would comfort me and tell me they were just dreams, I couldn't shake the feeling that they weren't, and I was almost always right.

I knew what was going to happen before it did. I could see and hear things that didn't make sense, and despite the loving environment I had at home, I felt totally lost, frightened and alone a lot of the time. As a result, my self-confidence was non-existent, although again, I was great at pretending otherwise. Life took many turns, and from a very young age until my late thirties, I went through many traumas.

Big traumas. Life changing traumas; the kind that if left unhealed, would not only stay with you way beyond your childhood, but affect every decision you ever make in your future and that's exactly what happened.

In those years I went through abuse, suffered great loss, and my mental health worsened. My ability to pretend that everything was fine came in really handy, and often even those closest to me didn't know that I was struggling. Even some of my closest loved ones weren't aware that, at a couple of different points during that period, I seriously contemplated suicide.

But there was something inside of me that kept me going... a "wondering". It was the same sort of feeling as the hope I felt when I wished for clip-cloppy shoes as a little girl. An undiscovered longing for the person I hadn't yet allowed myself to be. And somehow, even during the darkest times, the call I felt pushed me forward; the call home to myself.

After an incredibly difficult few years, and with my mental health being at an all-time low, I woke up one day and decided that I had to do something to affect change. I didn't know what, I just knew that there was a better life available for me. I knew there was a different version of me waiting to be remembered, and I also knew that it was my duty to unveil it. So, I started.

I started with questions, and in the beginning, they sounded like this:

"How do you find out who you really are, when you're

deeply unhappy and can't even face getting out of bed in the morning?"

"How can you start loving yourself when you feel completely lost, unloved, unknown, judged and deeply misunderstood?"

"How on earth can you create an amazing life where you're not afraid to show the world all of your glorious wonder, when right now, all you can see around you is total devastation?"

The answer was relatively simple, it was the execution that was the biggest hurdle. But I now know that it's completely possible to transform your entire life by being authentically you, even if you have no idea who you are right now and it feels totally impossible.

What's even better is that the journey to finding yourself is filled with more unexpected magick and joy than you could ever believe! I know because I've done it, and what's more, I'm going to share some of how I did it with you so that you can set off on your own, beautiful, magick filled journey too.

We're all taught from an early age that society has norms and expectations, and that if we don't fit into them, then we should bend to ensure that we do. The problem is, if we bend to fit into someone else's version of what we should be, we are forced to shove pieces of ourselves into small, tucked away boxes and deny that those parts exist in the first place. As a result, we're creating versions of ourselves that aren't whole.

If you took the jam out of a Victoria sponge cake, it wouldn't be a Victoria sponge cake anymore; it would be an incomplete version that looks deceptively the same. It might still taste good, but it isn't the tasty treat that it could be.

The same applies to you; if you're denying or hiding any parts of yourself through fear, or lack of confidence, then you're showing the world a less juicy version of yourself when you could be smothering yourself in the delicious jam that makes you uniquely you, and living life as the most mouth-watering, deep filled cake in the shop!

To know yourself inside and out, to be totally authentic, to show up *exactly* as you want to, and create an incredible life full of everything that your heart desires, all you need to do is *not hide any part of You*. That's the easy part. There's no great secret or elaborate scheme, it really is that simple; don't hide! But to get to that point, you're going to have to be prepared to let go of who you are pretending to be now.

You're going to have to be willing to look at everything you believe, do, and say, and change it if you need to. You're also going to have to show who you are to the world. That's the challenge...are you ready for that?

The world needs you. It needs you to showcase your

authentic self so that more and more people are inspired and encouraged to show theirs too. You are here for a divine purpose, and knowing your own identity allows you to fully understand what that purpose is, and birth it into being!

So...here's my five-step toolkit for finding out who you really are. Not a watered-down version but the real, true, unadulterated and completely pure version of the person that you're longing to be.

Step one: Core beliefs

Without even realising, most of us fall into adulthood with a set of beliefs that we've inherited from our parents, or those who raised us. It's not necessarily a bad thing, but until I thought about it myself it didn't dawn on me just how much those beliefs can stop you from fully stepping into your own light. This applies to everything from small beliefs like how to behave at the dinner table, to bigger ones around topics such as love/politics/religion.

Think about the beliefs you hold around illness for example. When you feel unwell, what's your default setting? Do you tell yourself to get on with it and carry on regardless of how bad you feel because you grew up being told you mustn't have any time off, and must fulfil your responsibilities? Do you feel guilty for stopping and giving yourself the chance to recover as a result?

What about your beliefs about love? What have you been unknowingly taught about what love is and what it should look like? Do you expect your partner to act a certain way because that's what a relationship always looked like to you growing up? Do you fall into prescribed roles within your relationship because that's how it was for your parents? Are you happy within those guidelines, or are there things you'd like to change?

These are just two very basic examples of how we are all moulded into patterns that may not work for us. We tend not to see them ourselves so we carry on playing them out regardless, when we could be living and acting in a way that makes us feel much happier. There are so many areas to examine; politics, faith/religion, parenting, image... you name it, the list goes on.

I even examined the seemingly insignificant things like "should I have turkey on Christmas Day?" and more weighty beliefs and sayings like "blood is thicker than water". There is no right or wrong, everyone is different; that's why life is so rich and beautiful. If you're not living in line with your own beliefs, you're hiding your own unique beauty. When you start examining every area of your life, it can be scary to see just how many belief systems are inherited and not actively chosen. The wonderful thing is that it's never too late to make changes.

Re-assessing the bigger areas such as religion, relationship dynamics, sexuality, image, and parenting, for example, can feel difficult; any changes may affect other people and your relationships with them, so don't be afraid to allow yourself the time and space to get comfortable with any new discoveries you make.

Enjoy the process of getting to know yourself in this way. It's empowering knowing that you've examined these extremely important areas in your life and are now living in line with what you actually believe! Remember that this is an ongoing process, and one that you can revisit at any time in your life.

As situations crop up you get to decide what you believe and once you've started actively thinking about some of these areas, it becomes easier to see where you are out of synch with yourself. Start with anything, it doesn't matter what, and I guarantee that you'll be surprised at the results.

So, grab a pen and some paper, and start now. Ask yourself these questions and see where it takes you:

- What is my core belief around "x"? (choose a subject)
- Is this my belief or is it inherited?
- If it's inherited, what do I really believe? How does this make me feel?
- If I acted from this new core belief, would I feel more like myself?

Knowing that your core beliefs belong to you and aren't just passively inherited is huge, and it creates the perfect foundation on which you can build your true, and authentic identity.

Step Two: Boundaries

Knowing what you believe is one thing. Living by those beliefs is entirely another and can throw up some big challenges, especially if you've recently discovered that you need to make some changes.

Maybe you no longer believe that you should always help people no matter what the emotional/physical/financial cost to you. Maybe you're not happy to say yes to people all the time, and even though you find it hard to say no, you know it's something you have to do for your own mental health.

Deciding is easy. Putting it into practice, not so much. It takes courage, and if your self-confidence is low, it will take even more bravery than you might feel you have, but once you start, it will start to feel like second nature.

The example above happens to be one of the boundaries I set for myself. I still have to work at it sometimes because I've always been a "yes" person. I love helping people, but I used to help them even if it meant that my life became complicated or stressful as a result. In the end, it took a devastating life lesson for me to completely understand that you can't help everyone, and sometimes the best thing you can do for someone is to say "no" to them whilst *saying "yes" to yourself*. Don't get me wrong, I still love helping people. I love helping my friends and loved ones, and complete strangers too. In fact, weirdly, I do it every day as part of my work, but it's a choice that I make and not a default setting... and there's a really big difference.

Setting healthy boundaries is an essential ingredient to finding out who you are. Every morning when you wake up, you get to decide what and who you're going to allow in your life, and what/who you're not. Just because you said "yes" yesterday (if we use that as an example), it doesn't mean you have to do the same today, or tomorrow, or ever again! The most important thing is that you set boundaries that allow you to show up in life as you really want to. You can do it with everything. Re-assess, re-evaluate and re-write your own rule book!

There are some questions that help with this. So have a look below and see if you need to set up some new rules for how you wish to be treated and seen.

- What behaviors from others will I no longer tolerate?
- What daily routines help my mental health, and what do I need to set up in order to ensure I make time to do them?
- What stresses me, and how can I set new boundaries to minimise those effects?

- When someone/something upsets me, how do I want to react and how can I resolve it with as much ease as possible?
- What do I need to change about my day/time management to ensure I maximise my capacity?

Think about things like sleep patterns, screen time and finances as well as your interaction and relationships with people.

I found it helpful to journal all the new boundaries I wanted to set, and I urge you to do the same. Write them down so they become more real and a part of who you are. Say them to yourself over and over to break the pattern that you've followed previously, and to cement them into this newly remembered and empowered You!

Quite often, the people closest to us are the ones who find it harder to cope with belief or behaviour changes that we make. They know us as we are or have been. Personal growth means that previous ways of being changes, and that can be hard for others to get used to. It's important for you to know that the people who want the best for you will adapt and accept you exactly as you are, even if it takes them some time to get used to a new kind of relationship with you.

If you need to reinforce a boundary to someone in your life for the first time, do it clearly, concisely and from a place of love. Explain to them what it is that you're no longer accepting, and that, as part of your growth you hope they understand. Nine times out of ten, they will, but as anyone who has been through any kind of transformation will tell you, it's inevitable that you will lose people along the way.

Hold on to the fact that those who are meant to be in your life, will be, and those who don't will fall away. It's all part of the cycle of life, and it's better to be surrounded with people who want you to be the very best version of yourself and cheer you on, than those who pretend to. So be brave! Set those boundaries like a total badass, and step into a brand-new way of honouring yourself!

Step 3: Image

It seems kind of obvious, but the way you present yourself aesthetically has a massive effect on how you show up in life. How many times have you done your make up and thought "I wish I could wear red lipstick today" or, "I wish I had the guts to wear those leopard print trousers"?

(I'm using female examples, but the same ideology applies to men too)

How many times have you seen someone and thought "I'd love my hair like that" or "I wish I had the confidence to do that job"?

I'm not talking about wishing you were thinner, smaller,

taller or all of that kind of stuff, that's a different thing altogether. I'm talking about longing to wear the clothes that make your heart happy and not daring to in case someone doesn't like them, or not putting on your red lipstick on a Tuesday morning, because people might think you're too extra.

To me, it's like ignoring your soul when it's speaking to you, and that's damaging. Why not allow yourself to use your clothes, hair, make up and every outward aesthetic, as the creative expression of who you truly are? Some people will judge you anyway, even if you're head to toe in beige, so you may as well wear what makes you feel amazing and be totally you.

As Preston Smiles always says;

"Other people's opinion of you, is none of your damn business"

He's right. Plus, more often than not, we see that woman in the frozen veg aisle eyeing us up and down and automatically decide that she's being mean and judgmental. However, she may be thinking "they look amazing!". It's nowhere near as scary as you've built it up to be, that much I guarantee.

So, if you long to wear crazy trousers, wear crazy trousers. If you wake up one morning and want to wear a silk scarf that you bought years ago because you saw a woman with a head wrap and loved it, put it on. If you want dreadlocks, tattoos, or pink brogues, get them.

Listen to the voice of your soul, and nurture yourself by following it. It's liberating and an incredible act of self-love to show yourself through your individual creative expression, so stop playing small, and step out of the shadows!

Step four: Conscious Connection

It's no secret that I'm a total spirit junkie. I have very firm beliefs about what's beyond this physical world we have chosen to be part of at this time, and my personal conscious connection is very deeply rooted in all that I am and believe, but that doesn't mean yours has to be rooted in the same.

You can be totally connected and not be in any way religious or spiritual. In fact, you can be connected and not believe in anything at all.

Being consciously connected means that you are actively aware of how your body feels at any given time. Quite often you'll travel through your day without really checking in on how you feel physically. We always know when we feel sad, happy, angry etc., but how often do you *feel* into your body? Conscious connection teaches you to stop and reconnect with your physical body as often as possible, and it's a great way to make decisions too! Let me explain...

Imagine that you're in a situation where you need to make a decision. Take a moment to close your eyes and take a deep breath, then think about the decision you're trying to make. Imagine that you've already made a choice about which direction to go in, and as you do that, bring your awareness to certain centres in your body; your head, heart, stomach and sexual centre.

Concentrate on them one at a time. How does that decision make you *feel*? Does it feel ok in your head and heart but when you connect with your stomach, something feels uneasy? Or maybe it feels great in every centre except your heart? Whatever you feel, you must hear the answer and act accordingly. It takes a bit of practice if you're not used to doing it, but like everything it gets easier over time and soon enough, it'll become second nature.

If something doesn't sit right in all the centres of your being, then it needs looking at again. Knowing who you are is as much about learning to trust your body and listen when it talks to you. You've heard people talking about "gut instinct" before? Well your physical conscious connection is like a ramped-up version of that; bigger, better and always ready with the answers!

Step Five: Aligned Action

I've learnt a lot in the last 8 years. I've done a lot of reading, watched a lot of YouTube videos, listened to a lot of podcasts and been to many training/coaching sessions, but all the knowledge in the world doesn't mean anything at all if you don't use it.

The most important step in any program you ever do is making sure you take aligned action.

Not just once, or just for a week, but every single day. It doesn't matter what you have to achieve, or how far you have to go to reach where you want to be, if you don't take aligned action every single day, you won't get there.

This doesn't mean you have to have it all figured out now, far from it. Your belief systems don't have to be completely reassessed tomorrow, but you do need to start somewhere today. Setting those new boundaries so that you can start showing people what you believe in isn't something that you have to have all figured out in the next month, but you at least need to be working on them.

Deciding to find yourself through creative expression doesn't have to start with a total make-over right this minute, but maybe that wardrobe clear out you've been putting off is something you should make happen this week.

Look yourself in the eyes. Really see the person staring back at you, and promise her/him that you will take steps (it doesn't matter how small those steps are) of *aligned action* every single day to remember who he/she is.

You see, we can all hope for clip-cloppy shoes until the cows come home, but at the end of the day, until you -

1. decide you want them,
2. tell the woman in the shoe shop that you won't accept anything else,
3. be brave enough to wear them whenever you feel like it,
4. remember to think about how amazing it will make you feel, and
5. do what it takes for however long it takes to make all of that happen, you're always going to be in rubber soles...wondering.

I know you can do it, because I did. I still am, and my hope is that this goes some way to helping you discover your own, very special brand of magick!

*Magick = magic that happens as a result of spiritual practice or acts of radical self-awareness

AUTHOR BIO

CATE MCMURRAY

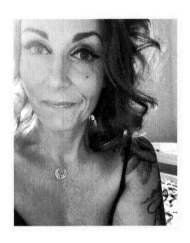

As a little girl Cate spent many hours picking up fallen rose petals and collecting rainwater from the garden of her childhood home to make magical rose water potions.

Little did she know then that her whole life would be filled with that magick every day. Not only that, but that she would then go on to help others who feel lost, find their very own brand of magick too!

Among those who know or have worked with her, Cate is known as a Spiritual Badass who is as authentic as it gets.

Her moral compass never waivers and her heart is full of love and compassion for all living beings.

She believes her divine purpose is to help people find their way back to themselves after suffering trauma and loss, teaching them how to foster a deeper personal connection to truth in every aspect of their lives.

With Cate's loving guidance people discover they can overcome any obstacle no matter how insurmountable it may seem.

Cate is a single parent who has Autism, as do her four children, and her experience of parenting whilst learning how to live with her own neuro diversity, has given her extensive knowledge of the many challenges this presents.

She has discovered the best strategies to make those challenges easier to deal with in the long run and will be the main speaker at a large Autism event in 2020, where she will be sharing her experiences with other parents who have children with Autism.

Cate is determined to help as many people as possible by using the ancient knowledge passed down to her by generations of Witches and her deep connection to Source.

As a thriving survivor of mental and physical health issues, including epilepsy and severe depression, Cate uses her many traumatic life experiences as a source of deep connection, empathy and understanding.

Drawing upon the wealth of knowledge learnt from her life situations, Cate teaches people how to create the beautiful life they deserve, no matter what they are facing.

She has helped many who feel lost back to their own path through her courses, one-to-one coaching, Goddess retreats and speaking events. She has also spoken about Witchcraft on BBC radio, and is currently writing her own book which is due to be published next year.

What else should you know about her? Well...she loves the moon, trees, and feathers and has a penchant for anything with sugar in!

Horses are one of her lifelong passions along with music, which means you'll often find her doing bad kitchen dancing...always barefoot, and sometimes (often) with a wooden spoon in her hand as a mic.

To work or connect with Cate, visit:

Website: www.catemcmurray.com

Email: cate@catemcmurray.com

facebook.com/catemcmurraywhitewitch

instagram.com/cate_mcmurraydotcom

7

CATH STOCK

IT'S ALL JUST ENERGY

*W*ell, who'd have thought that every single one of us has a 'sway'? No seriously, you have. It's a little-known secret I'm going to share that you can use to guide yourself.

If you don't believe me, pop the book down for a minute and try it...go on I dare you! You'll be amazed.

Stand with your feet about hips width apart, knees slightly bent, arms relaxed and your hands by your sides. Close your eyes and take 3 nice, big long deep breaths in and out. (Imagine your brain gets in a lift; goes down one floor; the door opens and brain gets out of the lift and chills out for a bit with heart...this takes you out of your head (where we sometimes do too much "thinking") to your heart energy and read what's REALLY going on).

Now say, your own name, "My name is ..." You will feel yourself sway slightly forward, indicating a "yes".

Say, "My name is Fred Smith". You should feel yourself sway slightly backwards, indicating a "no". This is what I mean by "your sway". If you have any resistance, I describe later in the chapter how to easily release this.

So, now do you believe me?

It's nothing weird or sinister; just an idio-response that happens automatically. If something is good for you, you would move forward towards it, right? And the reverse if something was harmful or dangerous. This is a very natural reaction to happen in our brains and bodies.

If only I had known that everything is just energy when I was crippled with depression, anxiety, panic attacks and losing the will to live, literally, and that it could all be released and transformed...and that the Universe really is there to love, support and guide us.

I will come back to the sway, how I discovered it and how you can use it to help you with anything in life, later.

I don't remember exactly when my mental health challenges first started...I do remember my husband, Tim, being very worried about me and begging me to go to the doctors, but I refused for a long time...I couldn't bear to admit I needed help... I thought that I should tough it out and get through it all...I believed that people would think badly of me if they knew.

I became more withdrawn from even my closest friends because I felt like I was failing, but I did manage to go with them to Pizza Express one night.

I wasn't feeling good...they were all talking about what their kids were doing...Both my teenagers (who I loved deeply, of course and still do with all my heart) were going through extremely challenging times and I felt a failure. My son had been temporarily excluded from school for having cannabis and was in trouble with the police for driving stolen cars under age and my daughter had been beaten up several times and was being bullied in and out of school.

This had been a huge shock for us both...we were just normal hard working, law abiding parents who thought we had done a good job of bringing our kids up...one minute we had these beautiful gorgeous little ones and boom...teenagers emerged like chrysalises breaking the skin and cocoon of early childhood and emerging...well, it's hard to describe how much they can change...It certainly wasn't what we'd expected!

I went to the toilet and was completely overwhelmed. Why me? It must be my fault. I should have protected Jody and well...Jake...Wow...I'm such a shit parent...and God, what if the parents at school find out...oh crap...no I mean really?

Me, a brand-new teacher in a high profile school, please God, don't let the parents find out...and what would they say if they knew I needed medication? What would they think of me teaching their kids when I can barely function? I needed time off school to go to court twice with him and felt so ashamed...but my friends' kids were doing so well, doing the usual things like going to school, clubs and achieving well with normal family lives...why is MY life falling apart?

It must be me because if I was strong enough, I would be holding it all together...that's what a good wife and mother does, they stay strong, well look at you, you're pathetic... I broke down completely, the panic gripping me so tight in my chest, heart, lungs I could barely breathe...

I text my friend, Linda, who knew what was going on and said, "I can't do this".

"Where are you?"

"In the toilet..."

"I'm coming down."

It was the start of over 20 years on and off medication, suffering from depression, anxiety, panic attacks and sometimes feeling suicidal.

The panic attacks got worse...I would feel totally paralysed and I remember sitting on the drive many mornings in the car or outside school in the car park, gripping the steering wheel so tight my knuckles turned that very attractive death white and my dry skin would split...my chest completely solid

I remember feeling totally overwhelmed with every part of my life...being a good mum, wife, daughter, teacher, sister (you get the picture?) and having those mornings when I just couldn't get out of bed because it was just too hard to face the world...it was just much easier to pull the duvet over my head and stay there, right?

Because I felt safe there...then guilt and self-loathing joined the pity party. Oh man, they love to kick you when you're down, don't they? ...lying in bed at night torturing myself because I felt so overwhelmed and I hated myself for not being able to cope with life, as I perceived others did.

Looking back and joining the dots...overwhelm kicked off panic and fear and anxiety and all that cycle of desperately destructive feelings and behaviours.

My life changed when I met this incredible woman in a purple dress at The mind Body and Soul Show in May 2017... I was completely transfixed by her and her group of people talking about "energy" and teaching people to "sway"!

IT'S ALL JUST ENERGY...FEELING STUCK...CHANGE YOUR LIFE...LAW OF ATTRACTION...really?

No, I mean, honestly? What the hell?

This is where I first discovered that neat little trick of having a sway!

I goose-bumped (bumped into each other and gave each other goosebumps) the amazing lady in a purple dress. I didn't know the significance of this at the time.

I'd been introduced to the Law of Attraction during my network marketing days and it was the first time someone had planted a seed that I could have a different life.

I saw all those people successful, happy and abundant in every area of their life and I wanted whatever it was that they had, even though I didn't know exactly what "it" was.

I realise now, I was actually studying the energy and I went to every training possible and followed what the leaders did to try and achieve that illusive Nirvana. I never cracked what "it" was but it led me to the lady in the purple dress.

The lady was Yvette Taylor and the energy "thing" she was doing was EAM, The Energy Alignment Method®.

She said goose bumps was an energetic sign that we were meant to meet and that I was on the right path.

That's what the lady said and before I knew it...

I agreed to go and hear her speak for an hour.

I signed up for a day course.

I signed up for a 10 month course.

I was so impressed by how it changed my life and so many others, I trained to become a mentor, so I could teach and facilitate transformations for others.

Day 1 of my first EAM weekend is where my journey started.

I knew I was starting something that would require me to dig very deep into myself, and I was afraid of what I would find. I was terrified about all the things I was hiding from, and where I perceived to be "failing" in so many areas of my life.

Walking over for breakfast, I felt the old familiar feeling of my old adversary, Anxiety and his best mate, Panic Attack taking hold...

As expected, everyone was lovely. We smiled and chatted and asking what it was we hoped to gain from the weekend? At that point I felt sick, the anxiety in my chest and stomach completely took me over inside. I walked back to my room, breathing heavily and crying, trying to pull myself together.

I argued with myself, I can't do this, yes you can, but it's too hard, but you NEED to be here, that's why you've come, but I can't, I really can't do this... Maybe you can identify with this, or know someone who suffers like this?

Eventually... I pulled myself together and forced myself back over to the main building. I was feeling horrendous. On arrival, Lisa welcomed me and asked me if I was ok? I just broke down. "No, I'm not...I'm just feeling really anxious..." Instantly, Lou, my mentor was there with an arm around me and took me to one side, giving me tissues, and reassuring me I was in the right place and all would be well.

That day, I had an overpowering feeling I didn't understand, a feeling that I had something big to release. I told Lou and we began working on it together; she promised me we could continue the following day. I woke in the night with a sensation that I was too scared to deal with on my own. I told Lou straight away in the morning and we worked one to one until I had a sense of a huge shift of that resistant energy.

As I sat quietly afterwards in the window ledge enjoying the peace and the light watching the world go by...I realised...my anxiety had gone. The space where it used to live in my heart was empty...over 20 years of anxiety and panic had completely disappeared.

That weekend, I felt so ashamed and embarrassed at first and then so relieved to find out I wasn't the only one to feel a failure, anxious, suffering from self-sabotage, this was HUGE; I genuinely thought I was going crazy and to discover I wasn't alone was so reassuring.

Thankfully, since I discovered EAM (Energy Alignment

Method), I no longer need any meds and deal with life's challenges using energy alignment and coming from a place of unconditional love and gratitude.

Don't get me wrong, life still throws me curve balls and I feel terrible but I can recognise it now and deal with it straight away, proactively. I bounce back quickly in a way I never imagined was possible.

Now, I put myself first because if I don't look after me, how can I help others and be there for my friends and family?

Finding EAM hasn't only changed but saved my life because I realised that my suicidal feelings were JUST ENERGY! Jeez...why didn't I think of this SOONER? Because everything comes in its own time.

So...this is how it works, in a nutshell...

Energy exists in 3 states, in flow, resistance and reversed.

Resistance is when you feel a push and pull between what you want to do or achieve, for example you may hate your job and want to apply for another one but you're too afraid to go and look for one because you dread the interview process. Fear is a heavy low vibration resistant energy that keeps you stuck. You might also be feeling anxious about moving jobs and depressed because you feel stuck, stressed and frustrated with yourself for not being brave enough to go for another job. All those negative, low vibration emotions are also resistance. I will come back to the job scenario shortly.

Reversed energy can be caused by something happening that you're not even aware of that causes your energy to go into shock and break off or just get stuck, energetically. For example, you might be afraid of teenage girls because you were bullied at high school. By asking your sway we can clarify when it started, and it might have been when you were 5 you were walking home from school with your mum and some teenagers jumped out at you scared the life out of you.

By asking your sway we find out what is going on in your energy because we all have an aura that records all our experiences and stores our memories.

In flow...this is what we all want, isn't it? You know those days where everything comes easily. You have no resistance to what you're doing and you're in a high energy vibrational state with emotions like joy, love, happiness, abundance. Your head, heart and hara (your creative and manifesting energy centre) are fully aligned and singing from the same hymn sheet!

We also use The Emotional Scale as a very useful tool. Put simply, if you drew a horizontal line, this would be the baseline. Below this line are all the heavy, resistant, slow, heavy vibration emotions such as guilt, depression, anger, hate, anxiety etc and fear which is right down at the bottom. It literally keeps people stuck from moving forward in life. Because like attracts like, many people stay trapped in cycles of these negative, destructive cycles, just attracting more of the same.

If we can begin to release these and come up to the neutral line, we can then transform and bring in high vibration emotions such as peace, happiness, joy, hope, love. These are high vibration energies, which then attract more of the same. Unconditional love is the highest vibration energy right at the top of the scale.

So EAM works by us being able to release low, heavy, vibrational energy and transform it into high vibrational energy.

If you imagine your life, experiences and memories are full of balloons of resistance, each time you release it, you clear one; it's like popping a balloon and letting it go. There are still more to pop, so you keep going and every time you burst one, you release low vibration energy. The more high vibration energy you bring in, the more you attract.

So... the steps to using EAM, in brief, are...

Step 1 you ask a question.

We always do this work out loud because we need to use our voice energy as well as our heart energy.

Always use your name as a guide question first to make sure your sway works.

Let's use the scenario of wanting to apply for a new job.

Get yourself into the sway position and think about applying for a job, going for an interview etc.

Ask the question out loud: Am I afraid of applying for a new job?

Step 2 You move forwards or backwards Y/N (Yes/No)

Step 3 You experience

Focus on the emotions first. You can write these down and ask your sway how you are feeling? Eg fear, anxiety, like I might look a fool, scared of being rejected, fear of being judged?

Question:

Do I feel anxious? Y/N

Do I feel scared of being rejected?

Do I fear being successful?

So, you might have learned that you are anxious, fearful and scared of being rejected.

Now focus on your energy; where or how you are experiencing that in the body? It might be a hard, red ball in your heart that is like a burning fire; or like a glass wall around you.

Everyone experiences their energy differently.

Step 4 Release and transform

We stand with our eyes closed, in the sway position and say clearly, out loud:

"I am ready to transform this hard, red ball in my heart that's like a burning fire that makes me feel anxious, fearful and scared of being rejected. I release it from my energy in all forms, on all levels at all points in time". Take a large deep breath in and blow out the longest breath you can. Take another 2 similar deep breaths in and out to blow the resistant energy away.

Repeat this statement and 3 long breaths in and out 2 more times.

Let the energy settle by just staying still and focused for a minute and then reassess and check in with your body to see how your energy is feeling.

It's important to do the statements 3 times to address every layer of our energy and to create and strengthen new neutral connections in the brain.

Focus back in the sway position and see what it feels like now? Can you feel anything left? Has it gone completely or is there, for example, a tiny warm red speck that you can sense still in your heart? Check with the sway, is this small red speck still resistant energy that makes me feel anxious and scared? Y?N

If it needs another release, repeat the above step 4 statements and procedure 3 times.

Then check in with your energy. If you think it's all gone, ask the sway, "Have I released all the resistance?" and "Do I still carry that resistant energy?"

It's important to make sure you have released all the resistance before you do step 5.

Step 5 Manifesting/creating what you want to experience

I call this creating a recipe from the Universe of what you would really like to experience and feel now around the subject you're exploring. It's important to take your time to write down exactly what you want to manifest/bring in and before we say the words, the energy state we are in is vital to bring in the highest vibration energy possible. Remember, like attracts like. The more high vibration energy you bring into your life, the more you will attract!

If we take the example of releasing all the fear and anxiety-based resistance as well as the beliefs of not being good enough, you now are free to fly! Get yourself into the sway position with your eyes closed and imagine what it's like being fearless and full of confidence in yourself to apply for and smash your job interview to get the perfect job!

Like we did with step 3 resistance, see what this incredible energy feels like and where it is for you? Is it inside you/outside you? What shape is it? Does it have a colour? Is it still or moving? How big is it?

For example, it could be an incredible gold ball around you, moving and swirling. If it's just outside you, expand it to fill the room; swirling and lifting you up to support and guide you.

Make that bigger and more vibrant and stronger still till it fills the world and you feel invincible. Imagine it filling every layer of your aura, so you are fully expansive.

At this, point, you have increased the high vibration energy to the biggest and most powerful it can be, you are ready to say the step 5 statements.

You get in your sway position, with your feet slightly further apart. This time you put both arms up in the air above your head as wide as they will go with your fingers closed; hands pointing upwards.

Then say out loud, "I am ready to allow/receive/align feeling more than worthy and I KNOW that the perfect job comes to me with ease at the perfect time. I speak with confidence and flow and my new job provides the perfect work life balance for my highest good. I welcome this into my energy in all forms, on all levels and at all points in time".

Repeat the 3 breaths and statements a total of 3 times

and on the 3rd, bring your arms down slowly to bring the energy in.

Wow! How different will you feel now about getting a new job?

Isn't it amazing that we all have the power within us to transform our own energy in any situation?

If ever your sway isn't working, you can just use the releasing statements to release any resistance eg "I'm ready to release and transform any and all resistance to my sway working" and do a step 5, such as, "I'm ready to align to my sway working perfectly."

My life is so different now; still bites me on the ass! I cry shout, spit my dummy out and swear at the Universe (a lot! No, seriously I do, "What the heck...why me?") ...but I use EAM to release, transform and recalibrate my energy. My "bounce-back ability" is so much quicker because I have changed the set point for my emotions, thought, feelings and beliefs so I am operating at a much higher level of high vibration energy.

I eat, sleep and breathe EAM as a lifestyle choice. If I keep it up, I'm more than fine! I'm happy, healthy, calm, with so much more certainty and confidence; belief, trust and faith in myself and the Universe. And I notice a huge difference if I don't; my life just doesn't flow and the little things (and big things) get to me and I start feeling the old paradigm thoughts, patterns and beliefs full of overwhelm and anxiety.

I have a choice every day to start my day with an EAM routine that's like brushing my teeth, and every time I get challenged by anything or anyone, I stop and use EAM.

EAM is a free, simple tool that anyone of any age, background, ethnicity, sexuality, ability or disability experience can use.

I thank you deeply from my heart for being open enough to read this chapter. The Universe really loves and supports you; it's no coincidence you picked up this book.

You have the power to create the transformation yourself, you HONESTLY do...All you need do is make the decision. Are you ready to let go, to move forward to create the incredible life you were meant to live and set free the awesome person you are; that beautiful soul?

And remember... you REALLY do have a sway! It's all just energy. You don't need anyone else to change your life.

You already have the power and magic within, deep inside you. Its time to let it flow.

AUTHOR BIO

CATH STOCK

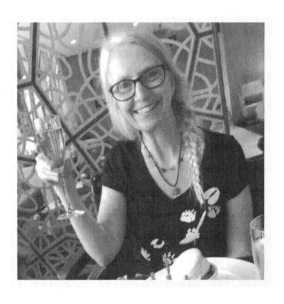

Cath is a mum of two and has two gorgeous grand-children.

As a mature student, she obtained a BEd. First Class Honours degree and her background as a teacher and art specialists enables her to use a unique, creative and multi-sensory approach with clients to encompass the whole self.

She is one of only 31 people globally, currently trained as a mentor to work with people using EAM since it became fully accredited as a new ground-breaking holistic therapy in December 2018.

She is a member of The International Institute for Complimentary Therapists.

Her passion and key message is, "It's all just energy and every one of us has the power within to make the changes.

You have to sow AND NURTURE the seeds to create lasting transformations."

You can contact her via email cathystock@sky.com

You can join the free EAM 5 Days to Flow

https://yourimpact.online/eam/

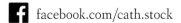 facebook.com/cath.stock

8

DANIELLE DOWNEY

*W*ho you are, at this moment is not who you have to be forever.......
Your past was a life lesson and not a life sentence.

Bold statement's hey?

In a nutshell, your past does not have to define your future. You have a choice about how your story will play out and who you will become. You are the master of your destiny and the Spielberg of your movie. And, you can make the choice to make a change at any given point in your life. I promise you, it's true and I am living proof.

I've meet so many professional and successful people who feel lost, alone and hollow. Despite their apparent outward successes and wins they ask themselves 'is this it?' They are alive yet feel less than whole. They breathe and only exist. They are not living with intention, breathing deeply and taking in the beauty that is their life.

Maybe this is you? An achiever, a high performer, top of your game, BUT, and there is a but because you know there is so much more to you than promotions, pay rises and certificates, you just don't know where that bit lies.

You 'should' feel happy and grateful. Other's look at your life and from the outside see your successes and achievements. What they don't see is that 'busy' is your form drugs and alcohol. Being busy means you don't have to sit and think, to sit and ponder on the loneliness that you feel, despite being surrounded by people.

On the worries, the anxiety and the emptiness. On the events of the past that may be weighing you down, holding you back and feeling like a noose around your neck. Maybe they are hugely traumatic events; a bereavement, divorce, debt, health issues. Maybe you feel that they are seemingly smaller, insignificant things which others feel shouldn't hold you back, yet they hold significance for you. Maybe they have become you. All encompassing, holding you tight like weeds in a pond, stopping you from surfacing and breathing clean, pure air.

You rarely sit down because sitting down, slowing down means only one thing...... that you might just think! What if you start to think about your past, about the trials, the adversity, the hurt and the pain? What if such things surface and in thinking about them you fall apart, show weakness, shatter the illusion that you have painted for so many years and begin to unravel as you fall down the proverbial rabbit hole.

All of the above applied to me for around forty-three years. I thrived on being busy, on taking on more and showing the world how capable I was. My busy-ness defined who I was. And, I loved it. When people around me exclaimed about all that I had achieved alongside six small children and a career as a midwife, bringing new life into this world and then later as an Independent Domestic Violence Advocate, keeping the women at risk of murder or serious harm safe from perpetrators. Both jobs which I was extremely good at and passionate about.

I relished being part of something wonderful, which allowed me to help and empower women when they really needed it. Yet I still felt a failure, I had no idea who I was, what I wanted life to look like and where I was heading, except maybe to an early grave because of the amount of stress I was putting on myself. I never sat down. I was in perpetual motion and my mind never, ever shut off save for the blessed moment when my head hit the pillow and I was out like a light. That was until 06.42 every morning, on the button when I would spring out of bed and begin another ground hog day of being busy. I am frankly exhausted just recalling how I was back then.

I had always felt different and I know that it goes back to my childhood which was fraught with abuse, poverty and stress. My self- confidence has always been low and in childhood, desperate to put a stop to the nightmare of abuse and sadness I tried to hang myself.

Thankfully the noose broke, yet I remained low and struggled with feeling inferior to school friends. I was desperate to do after school classes, music lessons, dance lessons and not feel poor. I copied the other girls mercilessly, learning piano and ballet from them because it was something that I could never achieve for myself. And this my friend's is where I began to feel like an imposter. I had no sense of who I was and what I stood for.

The deep unrest and emptiness continued throughout my teenage years and on into adulthood. I was a clingy girlfriend, desperate for attention and desperate to be loved. I felt empty and often contemplated suicide as a way of not feeling the way I did. I didn't want to die, I just wanted to feel different and could not see a path.

I had little or no self-love yet expected it to be given by someone else. That seems so crazy now! Expecting someone to love me before I loved myself! I had little in the way of boundaries with any relationship and made some choice decisions that I am not ashamed to admit were pants.

On the face of it one might say then that for the first forty odd years of my life, my past, absolutely did define my existence, every single day!! And unbeknownst to me, I mostly allowed it to.

And on I bumbled, on a hamster wheel of activity, stress and angst. I was successful, an achiever on the outside with qualifications, experience and a job which made a huge impact positively to others, yet I felt hopeless, off balance and had no idea who I was.

As I reached my fortieth year I was diagnosed with an auto immune disease and began to look into the links between childhood trauma and health issues in adulthood. Research states that high levels of Adverse Childhood Experiences (ACE factors) predisposed sufferers to mental health and physical conditions.

Adults who had suffered one or more of the ACE Traumas were much more likely to have depression, drug and/or alcohol issues, cancer, stroke and suicide than the general population. I had scored very high on the childhood trauma stakes and suddenly it made more sense to me why my body was beginning to malfunction, why my mental health suffered and why I felt so different.

Coming to terms with my failing physical health, not being able to think, speak coherently, write, walk or even look after my kids was horrifically scary. I would often fall asleep for hours at a time, waking up to find the kids foraging for food in the kitchen. I put stuff in random places and couldn't remember basic information. I felt like I was dying! Being properly sick for the first time in my life made me reconsider how I was living my life and what else I could do to mitigate the sticky start I'd had, and the impact that it had had upon my body. I knew that I could not go on feeling less than whole and not being able to find joy within me.

When my doctor informed me that my symptoms were a side effect of my condition and that to some extent my past had predisposed me to a failing, ailing body and mind I refused to accept it. My past was not going to define me any longer. I have always been immensely stubborn and love to kick back and disprove statistics!! And so it began.

Change came slowly for me and I began to assert some boundaries into my life for the first time. With boundaries came the negative assertion from others that I was changing. I once read that Newton's third law in physics states, 'that for each reaction, there is an equal and opposite reaction'.

Whilst he may have been considering this from a scientific perspective this statement could not have been truer for me. I was putting in boundaries and those opposed to them pushed back harder, labelling me difficult and prickly.

With the boundaries came a new-found freedom, a voice which I had never encountered before telling me that I was worthy of respect, of love and of happiness. The voice came from deep within me. It was strong, forthright and deeply knowing about what it was that I needed. I believe that it was my gut intuition telling me that life could and should be different.

I had always used my gut instinct to keep me as safe as possible as a child, yet over the years I felt like I had lost contact with it. Disconnected, so to speak. I found that the more it awoke, the more powerful it got and the louder the voice became. It was like a positive feedback cycle. The more I listened to how I felt deep inside about decisions the more I learned to trust. The more I learned to trust the stronger the feelings got.

I can only describe the changes which came about after I began to assert my boundaries as revolutionary, life changing and all encompassing, like a tsunami taking hold.

I began to put in other changes into my life which felt good. For the first time in forever I took time out for me! I became less of a people pleaser and began running on the hills near to where I lived. My lungs burned, my legs ached yet I found the space and solitude magnificent. I began to take more notice of my body, noticing that my mind became quiet when I ran. I ran without music and took in the sights and sounds. I had none of the household chaos to distract me. There was no-one to shout 'wipe my bum' or ask me what was for supper or where a toy was!

Time and space on my own felt idyllic, yet so selfish. I

had spent so many years making my family the focal point of my day, of my very existence, that it felt alien to not be 'mum' twenty-four-seven.

These tiny, seemingly insignificant changes began to infiltrate my life and the overall effect compounded. I began to stop playing the busy hero and acknowledged and honoured my body when I felt tired. My thyroid disorder often left me listless with exhaustion with a brain fog akin to days of sleep deprivation. I became an expert in cat napping, discovering that twenty minutes allowed me an instant recharge. I took great delight in snuggling down with a blanket before the school run, setting my alarm for a decadent twenty minutes and snoozing. It felt rebellious and delicious.

And so, the changes continued. I began practising mindfulness using apps on my phone and good old YouTube. I listened to meditation in short bursts, often falling asleep briefly. I practised deep breathing, relaxation and took up yoga! I loved the pull of my muscles stretching and the deep connection I felt with the universe and Mother Earth when I practised my sun salutations every morning on my veranda. I felt as if my soul was awakening and as if every cell in my body was regenerating. I fell asleep muttering gratitude's to myself, like an ancient incantation and awoke thankful for the breath in my lungs and for my life.

My mood lifted. It was as if the fog began to clear from

my mind. My brain looked for the positive in every scenario and even when catastrophes struck, I felt calm. I am not saying for one moment that I didn't feel hurt, anger or frustration. I just began to realise that these were emotions or feelings. They didn't have to define my day, my week or even my being. They were merely states which I could control, because I was in control of me.

One of the smallest changes which I began to make and the one which has had the most impact was in starting a daily gratitude journal. Speaking out loud the things that I was grateful for felt powerful, however writing them down was doubly powerful. A study by Robert Emmons in 2003 found that participants who wrote down gratitude's slept better, exercised more and had lower levels of depression. I noticed that my aches and pains were less, they were easing and that I smiled more. My mood was enhanced, my thoughts clearer and my mind quieter.

Early on in my journey I began to reflect upon my past and the way it had shaped me. It would have been all too easy to focus upon my upbringing as an excuse for feeling lost and unhappy and to seek solace in alcohol or use drugs to numb my pain. I realised in my twenties that I had an addictive personality and thus made a conscious decision to steer away from drugs and alcohol as I realised that I had the propensity to become dependent very quickly.

It was within this reflection during my forties that I

began to realise that being busy was my drugs and alcohol. It was my self-destruct button and my crux. If I remained busy, I need never think about my childhood traumas of sexual abuse, isolation and loss.

Within my gratitude journal I began to feel grateful for my past experiences and I started to list all of the experiences that had given me a huge level of resilience, grit and tenacity. I would never have had such a 'can do' attitude, had it not been for my childhood. I still believe that there is little I cannot accomplish and am happy to learn a new skill in order to complete a task. I would not have a blatant stubbornness to get shit done, a refusal to give up and an enormous need to challenge unfairness. None of these attributes would have come from an easier start and for that I was wholly grateful.

I began to surround myself with like-minded people. I noticed the more positive that I became the more the negative people commented upon how different I was and on occasion how much it annoyed them! By then putting in place boundaries had become a habit. It became easier to limit the amount of time that I spent with them or in extreme cases close the door on the friendship altogether. I must add, I didn't feel that they were wrong and that I was right. There was no judgement on my behalf.

Many of us have been indoctrinated to believe that when we make decisions of such magnitude and choose to remove ourselves from relationships which do not serve us that we are bad people and perhaps should work harder to understand the other person and change ourselves. This of course is rubbish. We are always allowed to make and honour decisions which feel right for us at a core level. When we begin to trust our gut instinct and care less about societal pressure to conform, I believe that our lives become richer for it.

In shedding the friends who no longer served me I felt lighter, brighter and attracted new friends who wanted to also develop themselves and live their best life. It was as if in closing one door it allowed another to open.

These changes weren't all easy. Change rarely is. I was tempted to go back to the things I had always done, to take the path of least resistance, to go back to what I knew was warm, cosy, familiar. The friendships with friends who wanted to moan when I was having a bad day, the insidious negative thinking which sought to point out the bad in everything and the lack of self -love. All so easy to do, yet hard habits to break. It took practice and energy, focus and determination.

So, you may ask, was it worth it?

I will always reply HELL YEAH!

However, if I am honest, I am still work in progress. I believe we are never the finished article. Once we start on our journey to be the best human being that we can be we evolve and move through our life easier and change becomes less challenging.

So, why share this period of my life with you? You're in a good place, right? You are successful, passionate and love your life.

And, if that's the case then I salute you with both hands and with all my heart. You are where I dreamed of being for so many years. In a good place, where you live with intention, trust and self-love.

Yet, if you're not there 'YET' I speak to you.

To say that you CAN change, things can change and that you can be so much more than you believe at this moment in time.

Your past doesn't have to shackle you. It doesn't have to define you. You are not IT in its entirety. Your past was your lesson, your opportunity for learning, your chance to grow. That is all you need to focus on. You are in the here and now, with the chance to draw a line before all that has gone before you and move off in a different direction towards a life where you choose how your future will look. You get to choose how your personality will develop, what your habits will be and how you will spend your time.

In that respect it sounds easy doesn't it? Decide and do. Simples hey?

So why do so many want to change their lives and subsequently fail? Why do so many people wake up on January 1st every year, write goals which they want to achieve and yet, by the 15th January have paled into insignificance. I believe it is because they underestimate the amount of effort it can take to make changes. They underestimate how hard it will be, how tempting it will be to revert back to the more comfortable ways. They underestimate the time it will take and want the changes immediately! They want instant gratification and instant results.

They will label themselves a failure when they stumble. Some may then throw in the towel. They may decide that this path to a better life is too hard, too rocky, too bumpy and too steep. They forget and perhaps never capture how beautiful the view will be from the top of the proverbial mountain.

When we take the stress out of change and accept that we are infallible and have a propensity to go back on our intentions, regress and mess things up, we then free ourselves from the worry that we might fail. This way we can begin to change without pressure. With small, baby steps and a realisation that our past is not defining us any longer. We are not the sum total of our past. It was a lesson and not a life sentence.

My past certainly was one of stress, trauma, anxiety, violence, hurt, isolation, emptiness and sadness. I was fearful, tearful, full of self-loathing, manic, stressed, needy and a people pleaser. My past constrained and shackled me for over forty years and would have defined me forever had I not have taken the first step towards freedom. Towards a future which is mine for the taking and mine by design, as opposed to one dictated by my past.

Your past is never who you are, what you are and where you are going. You alone can decide to be free and live with intention. You are powerful beyond all comprehension and now is your time. So, take the step forward and LIVE boldly, LIVE loudly and with passion and feeling. Feel exuberant, feel free and reclaim who you are.

.

AUTHOR BIO

DANIELLE DOWNEY

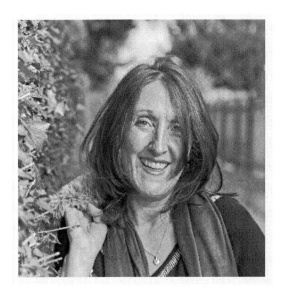

Danielle lives in East Devon with her husband and two younger children.

She is a qualified Life Coach with a recognised Diploma, a professional mentor and is a qualified Independent Domestic Abuse Advocate.

She is also a trained midwife and has a Master's qualification in Advanced Communication Skills.

In the past she has worked supporting and empowering women who have suffered domestic abuse to stay safe and make decisions which are right for them.

She has a studied conflict resolution and worked with clients with drug and alcohol dependency.

She is an Amazon Number 1 best-selling author with her own book, It's No Secret, Thriving After Surviving which was published in November 2018 and details her journey overcoming adversity.

She has been a contributing author in other best-selling books and has had articles published in online magazines.

She is a sought-after podcast guest, speaking about her determination to overcome adversity, her experiences of child sexual abuse and her refusal to let her past define her future.

She also record's her own podcasts interviewing exceptional and inspiring women who have a story to tell.

She has taken part in live events with The Survivor's Trust and is a staunch campaigner for the rights of women.

Danielle founded and runs a successful Facebook support group called Speak Out Sisterhood (SOS) which is a supportive community for survivors of sexual abuse and domestic abuse. It was founded because of her personal understanding of the importance of owning ones truth after abuse.

She is a finalist in the Blackmore Vale Business Awards in the Contribution of the Year Award for September 2019 for her work with Speak Out Sisterhood and was a finalist in the 373 Business Award in the Greatest Social Impact category in July 2019.

She works with clients in her transformational coaching business as The Rapid Transformation Coach.

She facilitates clients to live life on their terms and connect with who they choose to be.

She is an expert in empowering clients to put in boundaries, assess where they are and where they would like to be, make decisions which serve them and put plans in motion to help them to feel less stuck and lost.

A recent client quotes 'I am more confident in saying no and I feel like I am letting go of shit from the past and smiling more!'.

Danielle has a wealth of life experience to support her professional qualification's in coaching enabling clients to free themselves from a past which may not serve them.

She works compassionately and supportively via Skype or face-to- face at her seaside retreat in Devon.

In her free time, she enjoys running, reading, singing and is an avid writer ploughing away at her first fiction novel.

Contact:

www.danielledowney.co.uk

danielledowney40@gmail.com

https://www.linkedin.com/in/danielle-downey-9b428b109

facebook.com/danielle.downey.9803

instagram.com/crazykids

9

DEBBIE HAYES

RE-CLAIMING YOUR SELF WORTH

*W*hen life throws you a curve ball and all hope seems lost, my intention is to provide a lantern of hope to guide you out of the darkness.

Over the years people always told me how they saw me as the "The strong one", "Formidable", "A force of nature", "So positive".

Yet in 2018 I felt utterly broken; far from strong, far from positive.

I found myself in a situation so extreme, so abusive, so toxic. All the love, support and compassion I'd shown; thrown back in my face. I could barely breathe, barely speak. Tears streamed down my face, my body trembling, as I shared what had happened.

But it took months for justice to be serv ~~~~ longer for me to heal.

If only I'd listened to the whispers of my when those little things didn't quite add up or something just felt "off", instead of falling for a trail of broken promises.

Had I not endured enough in life? Another wake up call, seriously? I already felt as though I'd got a PhD in the University of Life. But clearly there was something I had missed.

Everything felt so unjust, so unfair. I HAD to break this pattern.

WHY, just WHY, WHY, WHY had all of this happened? Why would anyone treat me like this? My brain was searching for the answer. I HAD to stand up for myself and pull this "Weed" out at the root once and for all.

It really is the hardest lessons that give us the biggest blessings.

So, I went on my own personal quest to understand. And there I discovered some uncomfortable truths, some gems of wisdom and some lanterns of hope.

I reached out to trusted experts. It turns out that my empathic nature was like a magnet to narcissists who needed their energy supply. Through my research, I ınd out I had attracted this situation into my life. OMG! Two magnets with the same unconscious frequency of emptiness and unworthiness, both likely created in our formative years, but expressed in polar opposite forms.

Whereas I had an under-developed sense of ego and found my self-worth in learning to give, give, give; my polar-opposites had an over-inflated ego with a sense of entitlement to take and control. But they wore a mask of charm. And if this was ever questioned or the mask slipped, it would be met with a blaze of projection, belittlement and blame.

Wow, with this explanation, it all started to make so much sense. I'd experienced these narcissistic characters before, but this time it was on a whole new level.

I don't know if I was born an empath or whether it was a skill I had learnt. But it hit me in the pit of my stomach that as a child I had become an expert in reading the room, learning if I dare speak at any given point. I was "good" if I was "seen and not heard", "out of the way" and never daring to step out of line. Anything less wasn't good enough. That was fairly standard practice in the 70's. Speaking out, giving my opinion, asking for what I wanted, only ever seemed to cause anger and upset.

I learnt to silence my Self.

To never ask.

To never think about what I wanted.

To never answer back.

To never expect anything of anyone.

I learnt to be respectful, considerate and loyal. But now I see it was also a loyalty to neglect, to fear, to repression.

I silenced my emotions.

Buried them.

All of them.

The fear.

The tears.

The longing to be loved.

I was numb, empty, lost, so disconnected from my own needs.

I'd learnt all too well to be the "good girl". Not to let others down. This was the platform I had launched my life from.

As the years went by, people taught me to "Get on with it", "Not to rock the boat", "Try harder, do better", "Be more patient". You know the type of phrases I'm talking about. I continued to suppress pain, numb my emotions, "Pulled myself together" and became "More positive". That's how you deal with things right?

These reflections hit me like a lightning bolt!

I had often been told, "You get back what put out into the world" and I had taken this to mean my actions or positivity, but NO; these were just acting as a life jacket, serving to keep my head above the water.

What I needed to give out was a beacon of worthiness. Yet I'd spent 48 years emitting a silent beacon of suppression and sacrifice. Geez, 48 flipping years, am I a bit slow on the uptake or what?

I was a coach, I was known as "The Queen of Clarity", as it was so easy for me to see where other people were blocked. I knew all about beliefs, neuroscience, inner child work, the Law of ttraction, I had a fascination with metaphysics. But still I hadn't connected these dots.

In my own moment of clarity, I realised I'd been sleep-walking through life. I hadn't been consciously aware of this deep-rooted unworthiness. I had memories of previous traumas that had happened in my life. I thought I'd "dealt" with them. However, this emotional trauma had still been bubbling away under the surface, still stuck in my nervous system. So of course, its magnetic force had still been in operation.

All the jigsaw pieces started to come together. So many times before, challenges had come along to try and wake me. Some rather forcefully too. It seemed the universe stepped in and presented me with a whole spiral of events. Events that my mind interpreted as though they were there to tear me down; another layer of crap, another unjust link in the chain. But they were presented to make me stand up for myself. To say "No!", an invitation to cast off all the conditioning and finally see, understand and feel my value.

So, no more suppression, no more holding it together, no more pushing through. This time, I knew I needed to take a new approach, to face these emotions, to dredge the swamp. The decision was made. I was determined that I was NOT going through this shit again! EVER.

I allowed my soul to guide me. Gosh what patience she must have, I'm sure she secretly must have wanted to shout, "Please make a U-Turn" or maybe even, "For goodness sake woman, when are you going to listen and trust me at ALL times, will you just quit with the testing me out shit"

I was on a mission to clear this energy, I re-decorated the house; changed furniture, and burnt hundreds of sage sticks to shift the energy in the house.

I turned to an amazing EFT practitioner (Emotional Freedom Technique, more about this later) and a fabulous Reiki Master (who also gave me Bach flower remedies) to dig deeper, to allow things to surface and soothe my scarred nervous system, to ride the crest of the waves and go through the eye of the storm. No stone was going unturned!

I used several of my own coaching tools (gosh I was thankful for them!), took up offers of help, honoured my body's yearning to rest, heal, sleep, cry, even to FEEL; to feel lost, terror, anger, sorrow, the flow of tears streaming down my face, my heart creaking with stabbing pains.

There were days when I felt as though life was hanging on by a silk thread, a situation would trigger the tsunami of emotions and it felt as though I was right back at the beginning, dredging the swamp AGAIN. All the clarity and clearance I thought I'd got, seemed to be lost in the deep murky waters. All the confidence I had built seemed shattered. It stank!

I'd look in the mirror and wonder "Who are you? Your dull aging skin, your puffy face, your bloated belly". The cocktail of stress hormones was having far reaching impact on my lymph system, adrenals and thyroid. My health was in tatters. I had to look at this stranger and face who I had become; a shadow of my former self. It almost felt as though I was trapped in someone else's body.

Where was the spark? It had to be there somewhere, and of course it was, a flickering ember buried, buried deep under the layers of crap. I could see that deep inside, my soul never stopped sparking, she never gave up on me, guiding me to hang on in there.

I started to sense that parts of me wanted me to sit and listen, so I began to journal; asking the different parts of me what it was they wanted me to know, to understand, to acknowledge.

I developed a technique which I now call **Me, Myself and I.**

When speaking to Little me I would write with my non-dominant hand using a pencil; my writing so childlike. When speaking to my Intuition or what I now like to call my Inner-Tuition/my Soul I would write with a special pen. I would start by writing:

Dear Little me/Dear Soul what is it you want to share with me today..........

It's amazing what comes to light when you slow down and take the time to listen. And then I would journal with my adult Self, about what action she could take to address what had been shared.

My Little me would ask if I could just hold her, tell her that she mattered, that she DID count for something.

I allowed her to speak up, to talk about whatever she wanted:

"I just need to be held, I just need you to hear me, to feel as though someone cares. I just feel as though, nothing I ever do is good enough for anyone, I feel crushed, pushed away, worthless. Why are people like that, why are they so mean? I just feel so sad."

I heard her cravings to be acknowledged, nurtured, encouraged. I felt her pain and told her how much I loved her, how sorry I was that she didn't feel understood, and reassured her that I was here for her now and that we got through it.

I still feel so grateful that my Little me, felt able to share this with me. I now had the chance to tell her the truth, to say how wonderful she was. How I saw her brilliance, how I loved her unwavering determination and spirit, how amazing she really was, that she COULD reclaim her worth and shine out. She could speak, speak up, speak her truth – loud and clear. That I would be here ready and waiting to listen, to acknowledge her, ALWAYS.

When I journaled with my Soul: If I slipped into thinking that, I just wanted to "get back to normal," she would remind me that it wasn't a good strategy. Backwards was not the direction I needed to be heading.

Through my journaling practices, I built a strong self-awareness with Me, Myself and I. So many answers were revealed to me in our "conversations".

Like the rest of the clearing journey it required presence, stillness and patience and often a box of tissues.

I had to learn to be vulnerable. Initially holding the tears back behind closed doors, as the saga continued, I realised I couldn't protect my son from seeing me in a state of brokenness anymore. He turned to me and said "Mum, remember: The greater the suffering, the greater the peace". I was so stunned that a 13 year old could share such profound wisdom, that I felt speechless, words failed me and instead I just felt an enormous sense of pride. I always felt he was wise beyond his years.

Later, I asked him what he meant. "Well think of Auschwitz mum, when that happened, the whole world became aware of those horrific acts, and hopefully that will never happen again. Hopefully in time we can help other people".

That gem of wisdom did two things: It reminded me that although life felt awful in that moment, so many people had endured even worse traumas. But it also made me realise that my own suffering could be profoundly powerful and offer the world (potentially) the opportunity to raise its awareness and thus profound healing; a new way of thinking and a new way of being – for people to find a sense of inner peace, knowing their worth. It was one of those defining moments in life.

It gave me such a strong sense of clarity and purpose, a new sense of determination. I had to carry on and find peace with all that had gone before.

With the aid of the ho'oponopono prayer, I was even able to say thank you. Thank you to the universe for sending me the people that would awaken me, thank you to each soul that I had entered in to "Soul contracts" with to bring me these lessons. I'd used the ho'oponopono prayer previously, and wasn't too sure of its effectiveness. But something called me to revisit it.

I came across a YouTube clip with Dr Hew Len who explained using the prayer "I love you, I am sorry, please forgive me, thank you" by speaking to your inner child. This created such a shift, I got it on a whole new level, I could feel its power.

Through further research I learnt that the soul lesson for this narcissistic abuse was to help me acknowledge my courage and compassion. That my sense of unworthiness, could now be replaced with a growing sense of self-respect and self-love.

In many ways I wish I had chosen an easier "syllabus" but they say the universe only sends you what it knows you can handle, and clearly my Soul trusted that I was good enough for the challenge.

Intrigued, I had my birth chart read and was told my purpose was to "help people out of the darkness" that my life "Spoke to it" – WOW! I really was born into this situation.

All I needed to do was own it, I could feel my warrior spirit rising!

It was time to choose courage over control.

YES, people were right, I am strong, formidable, a force

of nature, I am so positive. So positive that I am worthy, that I AM ENOUGH!

I developed my warrior mantra

"A-Z of Enoughness"

I am Amazing enough

I am Brave enough

I am Courageous enough

I am Decisive enough

I am Energised enough

I am Fierce enough

I am Grateful enough

I am Heroic enough

I am Intuitive enough

I am Joyous enough

I am Knowledgeable enough

I am Loveable enough

I am Magnificent enough

I am Noble enough

I am Optimistic enough

I am Powerful enough

I am Quintessential enough

I am Robust enough

I am Strong enough

I am Thoughtful enough

I am Understanding enough

I am Vivacious enough

I am Wise enough

I am eXtraordinary enough

I am Youthful enough

I am Zealous enough

I would chant it out loud, and tap it in using EFT. I placed a crystal in my pocket and each time I felt it, I would repeat my A-Z to infuse the energy deeper and deeper.

You'll find more technical explanations about how EFT works, but here's how I like to think of it: We each have electrical circuits in our energy body. Our thoughts and emotions run through these circuits creating memories. These memories have an energetic charge which we store in our bodies. For example: You may recognise this as a knot in your stomach or a tightness in your chest.

When you use EFT by tapping on meridian points on the body you release negative emotions attached to the thoughts and thus restore your circuits.

The better the circuitry, the more energy can pass through and the more you SHINE. Hence it can be used to clear known "Blockages", i.e. illnesses, fears or worries or to release unknown "Blockages" that may cause us to self-sabotage when we tap in positive statements. Essentially it rewires any wonky circuits.

As my own energy rose, my Soul wrote this incredible visualisation in my journaling sessions:

You are The Warrior of your Soul

I invite you to step into your warrior energy, to truly emanate and percolate in that strength, that resilience and orientation to your highest Self, and allow it to step into every cell of your body.

Acknowledge him/her, apologise to him/her for abandoning that part of you.

Step into that brilliance, you are the warrior of your Soul. Feel that energy pulsating from your heart. Allow that energy to radiate out, feel the sparkling light emanating casting your brilliance and vibrancy further and further, you are the powerful creator of your life.

Notice the old worn out "clothes" of your previous Self on the floor, like an old skin you've shed. Imagine those "clothes" fading and dissolving into dust as a gentle breeze swirls and lifts away the dusty particles to be transformed by nature's wondrous rhythms.

You gently purse your lips and blow away any remaining specks of dust, they no longer serve you.

Your energy tingles with amazing light energy, you ARE the warrior of your Soul.

Your strength glistens, you feel so grounded and strong, so present with your magnificence, you feel the light shining from your eyes, beaming, you feel the pulse of your desires billowing from your heart.

You stand tall and proud. You are stood strong in your power, unhurried, present with your Soul.

Allowing this energy to deepen, to integrate, to be sooooooo familiar now.

This is You.

You are the message.

It made me tingle as I practised this. Within days, from nowhere people started to reach out to me with exciting new opportunities, to give talks, co-host a wellbeing radio show, even to write a chapter for a book to share my story. And here I am!

Yes, I did it! People were responding to my new frequency – YEY!

Thank you, thank you, thank you Universe.

Thank you to everyone in my tribe who has walked this path with me.

Thank you Me, Myself and I.

I love you and honour you.

I will listen to your wisdom.

I will act upon your guidance.

I will always allow you the stillness to rest, heal and restore your sparkle.

> **"Someone I loved once gave me a box full of darkness.**
>
> **It took me years to understand that this too was a gift."**
>
> **Mary Oliver**

Sadly, I know I'm not alone: perhaps you see parts of yourself in my story.

As I look around, I see numerous symptoms of people not feeling enough. Many people keep busy to avoid feeling the emotional gloop. Others create a showreel life on social media, but behind doors the reality is so different. Some people overthink things, questioning themselves and find it hard to make decisions.

When the pain becomes too intense, you see people turning to food, drink, drugs, exercise, anything that numbs and silences the very piece of them that so desperately wants to be acknowledged.

It's ok to feel. Once you allow your feelings to be expressed, rather than suppressed, it releases you. Accept and reclaim who you are, you don't need anyone's permission or approval and even if you had assigned them that authority, you would have given your power away. The sense of wholeness becomes your shield.

You can speak up and express your needs, set boundaries to ensure that your worth is never eroded again. To never get separated from yourself again.

If life throws you a curveball, it might just be happening for you, to show you what needs to be healed and reclaimed.

Trust you've read this book for a reason

Be courageous

Reach out to your tribe for support

Dredge the swamp

Allow yourself to be still

Notice what you notice

Journal using the "Me, Myself and I technique"

Practice forgiveness

Move forwards

Follow/create your own "A-Z of Enoughness" & remember to "tap it in"

Use the visualisation "You are The Warrior of Your Soul"

Invest in yourself, and keep increasing your value

BE A BEACON OF WORTHINESS

With Love Debbie x

DEBBIE HAYES

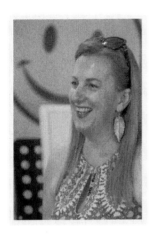

This photo was taken by James Byles in August 2019 as I gave a talk about "Creating Balance" at The Family Tree Wellbeing Festival.

When I saw it, it brought a tear to my eye, I was so pleased to see how it captured the sparkle back in my eyes.

Debbie Hayes

Clarity Coach * EFT Practitioner

TEDx Speaker * Author * Wellbeing Radio Presenter

Ambassador for Thriving post trauma and domestic abuse

Debbie holds over a decade of success in her coaching practices and a lifetime of experience that allows her to share potent words of wisdom.

She embarked upon her entrepreneurial journey in 2012 after having a serious accident which gave her the push to "Go for it".

Since then, she's gone on to work with large organisations supporting leaders and their teams to work together more effectively, run networking and coaching circles for women in business and help countless people when they've hit a crossroads in life.

Debbie's passion for coaching stems from the impact that it has had both on her own life and that of her clients. Having previously experienced and witnessed many others burn out, she went on a quest to change our working culture, supporting businesses and individuals to have the edge vs pushing them over it.

Recognised for these talents and for her unwavering stand for balance Debbie attracted an invitation to deliver her first TEDx talk in 2016. Her talk, "The true cost of being too busy", highlighted how our addiction to "busyness" is having far reaching consequences to people's mental and physical health and the erosion of communities and communication skills.

Debbie strongly believes that everything in life happens for a reason and that there is always a lesson in every situation we face. Her love of learning, practicality and spiritual inquisitiveness give her a unique perspective on life.

Debbie has an innate calmness and ability to hold people in a safe and supportive space. Her clients have awarded her the title "The Queen of Clarity" because of her intuitive ability to laser in on the root cause of their presenting issues with impactful questions. She's been told that her insights and tools deliver "life changing results" coupled with a true sense of fulfilment.

Never one to rest on her laurels, she's always open to learning something new that will further support her clients. Following the amazing results featured in this chapter when using EFT (Emotional Freedom Technique a.k.a. "Tapping") she decided to train as a practitioner herself, excited to share this transformative practice with her clients.

She loves life's simple pleasures; sharing good food with family, enjoying meaningful conversation with friends, walking her dog in the beautiful Cheshire countryside and taking trips to the beach. With a thirst for learning, you'll often find her with her head in a book, or journaling with her ever expanding collection of pens, sticky notes and notebooks.

Debbie's Passion: "Seeing people's souls sing and eyes sparkle again. There's no better feeling than to know you've helped clients believe in themselves; that they are good enough and can achieve and succeed in their goals."

Debbie's Favourite Quote: "Until you value yourself, you

won't value your time. Until you value your time, you won't do anything with it." – M Scott Peck

Debbie's Mottos: "Follow your True North", "Ditch the Popcorn Head" and "It's time to flick the dimmer switch and BEAM!"

Debbie's Words of Wisdom: "The greater the connection to yourself, the greater the courage to follow your calling."

When life throws you a curve ball never stay stuck or lost, reach out and say hello@debbiehayes.co.uk

Discover more details about how you can start your journey to joy by visiting www.debbiehayes.co.uk.

Download your free guide on how to use EFT (Emotional Freedom Technique) to tap in the "A-Z of Enoughness" complete with free poster and screensaver to act as an aid memoir at www.debbiehayes.co.uk/warrior

BREATHING

*H*ave you noticed that Breathwork is becoming a new norm?

Breathwork is the link between body and mind, between spirit and matter, between the conscious and the subconscious mind. The breath is a force, a bridge or a tool. It connects us to each other, and to our own nature, our source. It brings back the vital inner balance.

It is applied by more and more people across many industries such as the fitness, sports and peak performance industry, in the military, martial arts and medicine; as well as in psychotherapy, creative arts and corporate.

Breathwork has helped me tap into endurance running and aided me to process and release my early life trauma.

As an adoptee, I didn't realise I had any trauma, nor that it could be dissolved within my nervous system.

This is easy for me to say as a Breathworker today, however this wasn't always part of my belief system. Let me take you back to the start of my latest transformation;

December 2015: Bringing it back to the body, mind and soul

When I heard my doctor say burnout to me three years ago, it sent a shudder down my spine as I didn't fully understand what it meant. My initial thoughts were failure and shame, and my fears grew as I believed society would judge me.

The best way to describe my existence at the time was jailed in a life I never wanted. I lacked the tools, direction and self-knowledge, courage and faith to free myself, let alone any idea of what I might do even if I could escape. After accepting the word 'burnout' and not wishing to start taking medication I felt the need to change.

The hard part about change is not making the same choice. In 2016, I questioned everything and started my own journey of self-development and embraced change in my life. My change started when I listened to *Finding Ultra* by Rich Roll, a book I still do not know how it came into my orbit.

After listening to this book, I started to listen to Rich

Roll's podcasts, there wasn't much to catch up on as he had just started recording. Rich Roll interviews inspirational guests. In June 2016 I heard Wim Hof being interviewed. Wim Hof is also known as The Iceman by breaking a number of records related to cold exposure.

His feats include climbing Mount Kilimanjaro in shorts, running a half marathon above the Arctic Circle on his bare feet and standing in a container while covered with ice cubes for more than 112 minutes. He attributes these feats to his Wim Hof Method (WHM), a combination of frequent cold exposure, breathing techniques and meditation. I was intrigued and booked onto his winter Poland experience to learn more.

The Wim Hof Method explained

The Wim Hof Method (WHM) uses Breathwork training and gradually increasing cold exposure to influence your immune and autonomic nerve systems. Learning and practising the WHM allows you to overcome extreme conditions and supercharge your immune system.

The basic method involves alternating between deep breathing and breath holding. A simple yet powerful practice. With focus and commitment, you can learn to control your immune system and autonomic nervous system to improve your circulation, boost energy levels, improve concentration and focus, sleep better, put yourself in a more positive mood and take your performance to a higher level.

December 2016: Mount Snezka – the day I changed my mind

The Poland WHM winter travel experience ended with a mountain climb to the summit of Mount Snezka, wearing only shorts and a sports top. We did not make it to the summit that day due to terrible weather. Wim often quotes "nature is merciless", and although that day I could not control the weather, especially the freezing cold winds, my walking meditation allowed me to truly surrender as I naturally, and consciously, reconnected with my physiology to endure the harsh weather. I focused on the one thing I could control: my breathing, and - taking one step at a time - I surrendered to everything else.

Together, my mind, body and breath were focused in each step I took. It's a powerful state to be in when your whole body is acting as a single unit. The union gave rise to a different sensation (maybe it was the power of my mitochondria); every cell felt alive, combined with a quiet mind and a body that could cope; finally, a truly peaceful moment. It was a coordinated homeostasis.

I was empowered. It was the start of my new chapter.

January 2017: The Camino – the prelude to my self-actualisation

After my Poland experience, I wasn't ready to return back to my 'normal life'. Something had switched within;

a new pathway of thought. I felt the bliss of being and feeling limitless. These changes also opened my Pandora's Box and released my adoptee fears of abandonment. I intuitively knew it was time to process this.

I remembered a quote that stuck in my mind over the Christmas period, "When I was young, I was too busy, now that I am older, I am too tired." I did not want this to be me, a newly perceived successful member of society who was starting to transform in another way. So, I decided to continue my journey into the unknown and head to St Jean Pied de Port, the start of the French Way Camino. A 900 km trail, it is the most popular route to Santiago de Compostela in northern Spain.

I now know that walking the trail uncovers beautiful landmarks and hidden gems one step at a time. Being outdoors, communing with nature on a daily basis allowed change to occur within me. When I realised there was something missing, I became more curious to finding out what it was.

Every day of my pilgrimage, I realised that the nature I was seeing on my route was becoming more inspiring and was teaching me to break down my thought loops, and to 'let go' of what was no longer important to me. My mantra for the Camino was to live each day: 'Today is today and tomorrow is tomorrow.'

Each day, I adapted the WHM to my Camino. My cold exposures were either cold plunges in rivers, cold showers, or walking in shorts. I adapted my 'WHM breathing technique' for the Camino and tuned my body and soul (as I did on the mountain in Poland), harvesting my inner strength. So much so, I knew the weight of my rucksack so well I could tell if I was down to my last 150 gram chocolate bar.

In Pamplona my left ankle was swollen due to the weight I was carrying on my back. The next day, after a night of ankle elevation, I decided to start walking, my mantra for the day was 'breathe in love, breathe out hate', and I put my awareness on my ankle. By late afternoon I had caught up with the little group of pilgrims I had said goodbye to that morning. We had some olives at a bar and discussed what had just happened, I was walking well, and my ankle was not swollen.

Another poignant moment was when I was about to walk to Albergue Tomas in Manjarin. I was the last to leave our little group of pilgrims by a few hours, as I had stopped off in a coffee shop for the delicious chocolate churros.

When I arrived at the night's Albergue accommodation, I realised that—despite the delay—I had overtaken the pilgrims who had left before me, by at least an hour. It is not a race, far from it, but that day I learnt the power of Breathwork and flow state in more depth. It was that evening that a seed was planted: I could run an ultra-marathon like Rich Roll.

By continuing to connect to the WHM method every day, I became more conscious of my surroundings, my body and mind, my thoughts and feelings, and those of others. It took a snowy day in the mountains for me to realise that for too long I had abdicated responsibility for myself, always doing what other people thought was best for me. That day in the snow, I found my voice.

A Spanish pilgrim insisted I couldn't wear shorts in the snow. When I asked why, his answer was that while it was not illegal, it was too dangerous. So, I politely explained that pain was inevitable in life, but suffering was optional. In that moment, I took back control over my body, knowing that if I felt cold, I would wear over trousers, whilst he might have a miserable journey no matter what clothes he wore that day.

My last 'lesson' I want share with you: It took the gift of a plaster to open my heart and to start trusting in a way I never had before. I had a double blister on my heel and a Spanish pilgrim gave me a plaster, he was walking for three days with his friend, before returning back to his family and work nearby. He clearly didn't need plasters. He simply said he chooses to carry plasters for pilgrims like me. I finally understood the journey we are on is about compassion and being of service to others.

March 2017: Life is worth living *really* well

Back in Cumbria, I continued my connection with nature. I felt different, with more inner strength, connection and self-belief than I have ever had before; I had become comfortable in my own skin and now trusted my gut feelings.

I entered the Windermere Marathon and Lakeland Trails 55 km run, which is known as an Ultra Marathon. My excitement was less about placement; more about self-potential.

My only advantage was that I had cycled often around the 'honey pot' of the Lake District, so I knew the course well. The main problem was that I didn't really enjoy running; the furthest I had ever run was approximately nine miles, seven months earlier. I was secretly happy to have it confirmed that there was very little time to train the 'conventional way' for an endurance run. Upon receiving this news, I decided to train a very different way.

I made my training about aligning myself with nature's rhythms. It was about investing in myself, stepping outside the conditioned mind, cultivating self-under-standing and honing a positive mind-set. Part of my strategy was to pioneer new ways of feeling relaxed and to feel abundantly connected to my body and to nature. As ground-breaking as all the technological innovations in tracking apps and GPS watches may be, I found it more powerful to have a more primitive approach.

I knew from my experiences in Poland and on the

Camino that to soar I needed to look within. Deep within. I knew I could do this.

<u>How?</u>

I realised I would never give myself a hard time in regard to not putting in the 'conventional' distance or work. I would do daily natural cold exposure and explore breath retention and other Breathwork techniques including the Buteyko Method. This breathing method is also effective for asthma suffers. I also introduced daily Kundalini, Tantra and diaphragmic warm up Breathwork.

I connected with nature every day. I saw raw beauty in the tarns I swam in, noticing little details such as tiny glistening rain drops on the moss as I relaxed under a waterfall. The cold brings you back to the present moment. Hiking in the fells, passing shaded trees, brought me the delicious smell of seasonal wild garlic. Walking barefoot, I explored movement, climbing and hanging from trees.

I welcomed all weathers. On one occasion when the rain had ceased whilst I was swimming in a tarn, it soon restarted as I set off home. I had a beaming smile while cycling home as it was an extended cold exposure and I thought 'it is what it is'. My daily adventures were a balance of struggles and challenges, yet I felt alive as they rewarded me with more joy, more fulfilment and a sense of purpose as I explored and anchored.

I saw that everything was active in nature. I experienced this and I began to feel a part of this activity. Nothing can replace our raw self; surviving the outdoors and feeling alive, by truly challenging ourselves physically and mentally. This realisation pulls us to discover our potential.

The stewardship of nature and our environment begins with loving ourselves in nature and feeling our connection to it.

The cold exposure enabled me to grow to new levels of actualisation, glowing outwardly because of the positive feelings that had been lit inside. I was no longer living disconnected to my potential. I was training with a healthy fear for the outer edge of my current capability. In nature, time passes quickly, a flow state as you tune into your breath, your thoughts and listen to your body. The soul exhales and relaxes as all your senses awaken, because you become an integral part of the outdoors and allow yourself the freedom to be imperfect.

On the day of my ultra-marathon

I cycled 6.2 miles to the start of the race. As I had never run this distance before, I assumed I would be back in time for my evening waitressing job at 6 pm. By 4 pm it dawned on me that I would not make the start of my work shift, so I called my boss and said, "I am literally running as fast as I can".

Other than that minor oversight, my ultra-marathon opened a track to the centre of my soul and proved the benefits of this different approach to be an easier way to live my life by going with the flow.

Learning Breathwork spurred me to be a more conscious thinker with greater gratitude for nature, created a more natural movement of my body, and led me to improve my diet and to immerse myself back into a community.

Since my Camino, my Windermere marathon and ultra-marathon, I am now a certified Wim Hof Method instructor.

I now accept whatever happens. We all need to learn how to accept the unacceptable, forgive the unforgivable, tolerate the intolerable, get comfortable with the uncomfortable, and love the unlovable because I believe we all need to learn to take our finger off our internal emergency alarm button. During my intense transformational year, I realised that most of my problems could not be solved by triggering my primitive fight or flight response. With consistent practising of the WHM, I now recognise this response.

In society, most of us overthink things and try to get through life using only our own neocortex or intellect or mind intelligence. However, we have two other center's of consciousness waiting to be awakened and accessed. All together we have three brains: one in our head, one in our heart, and one in our gut.

With Breathwork, we can tap into all three brains and therefore be fully present, create deeper connections, make better decisions, and keep ourselves safer. First, consider that you have three breathing spaces:

Belly, Chest, Head: Active inhale

Let go: Passive exhale.

Belly: Breathing into the lower breathing space allows us to relax into the body, awaken our instincts, connect to the earth, and feel safe and grounded in our body intelligence.

Chest: Breathing into the middle breathing space allows us to awaken heart intelligence and intuition and to connect to everyone and everything around us.

Head: Breathing into the upper space allows us to awaken mental energy or intellect, and to connect to higher intelligence.

Let go: releasing tension and pain, and relaxing more and more. Wisely letting go conserves your energy, clears your mind, gives you sharper insights, enables you to enjoy the here-and-now, and helps you increase your love for yourself and others.

Start by focusing on the belly. Bring all of your attention and energy to the floor of the pelvis and breathe there. Breathe into your tailbone, your hip bones and perineum. It's a meditation as much as an exercise. Send your breath along with your energy and awareness to the lower breathing space.

Next, breathe into the chest and diaphragm area. Have the intention to open your heart and connect to everyone and everything around you. Feel the expansion from side-to-side and breathe into your back.

Then breathe into the head (or upper space). You are breathing up into the small delicate spaces at the top of the lungs. Your collar bones tend to move up toward your chin when you breathe in. Imagine sending and receiving breath energy through the top of your head. Have the intention to clear and quieten your mind and connect with higher intelligence and heavenly beings.

Then exhale naturally, with no extra force, and relax more deeply with every exhale.

Create a wave as you fill all three areas with one active breath, followed by a passive exhale. This is circular breathing. Do it to create harmony between body, mind and spirit—instinct, intellect and intuition. Do it to be fully present, to be clear, conscious, relaxed and 'alive'.

The more we practice conscious breathing, the more we become aware of our response to situations in life and we can apply Breathwork when we feel anxious, afraid, stressed, shattered, confused or in pain. This is when it counts and when relaxation makes all the difference.

I discovered that behind, under, or within all emotions is

pure life force energy, and I learnt to integrate this energy in very powerful, positive and productive ways. I believe that breath is the key to happiness, strength and health — it is worth mastering, because these powerful energies serve us and the world.

Enjoy your practice, and warm wishes on your journey.

Trust the process of change.

EMMA ESTRELA

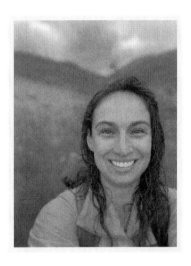

Living authentically - I thought I did until I heard Wim Hof on a podcast. His story resonated with me, especially that there is more to the Wim Hof Method (WHM) than ice and breaking world records. Science, Wim Hof's story and gut feeling drew me in. For me WHM has become a vessel to allow myself to truly connect within.

Applying the simplicity of the 3 pillars of the WHM,

this new inner balance has taken me to walk the Camino de Santiago in winter, wearing shorts, run my first Marathon and weeks later Ultra Marathon both in the Lake District National Park without any physical training. It has also allowed me to reflect where I have compromised myself and feel a paradigm shift in life's everyday emotional ups and downs.

I have experienced the Poland Winter Expedition both as a student and as an international instructor, this has expanded my depth and understanding of the WHM which is about knowing your own body and having conscious control of keeping it strong, happy and healthy. Do everything with clear and pure intentions and focus on the goal that is right for you. I'm excited to share this plus more of this powerful method with you and integrate it into your life too.

I live in the Lake District, a UNESCO World Heritage Site in the North West of England. Here you can connect with nature in my WHM workshops, one-to-one sessions, retreats and breathing sessions and I am willing to teach at private events worldwide.

Contact me to learn more or ask me anything about endurance running, early life trauma release, PTSD, anxiety, depression or the Wim Hof Method:

Email: emma@emmaestrela.com

Website: www.emmaestrela.com

LinkedIn: Emma Corrie

[f] facebook.com/emma.corrie.73

[o] instagram.com/Estre1a79

JILL TREVENA

PROACTIVE MENTAL WELLBEING
MATTERS

*D*o you know who you really are?...

Mental illness holds up every aspect of your being for close examination.

Mental illness is a tumultuous, often dark journey that throws you around and turns your world inside out. It challenges all you ever thought you knew. It draws out every flaw and fear. It forces you to dig the deepest you have ever been to find the strength to pull yourself above the surface.

Mental illness - I get it. I understand how it feels to be overwhelmed by anxiety, to be terrified and rooted to the spot with panic. To want to hide away yet at the same time feel terrorised by your own company. To feel physically sick, to be unable to eat or sleep. To struggle to put one foot in front of the other, to shower, put your clothes on. It's confusing and life altering.

This is my story.

I'll start by introducing myself as an occupational therapist with twenty years of experience in assisting people to manage their mental and physical wellbeing. I am also an occupational therapist with her own story of mental health challenges, and this is what I will share with you.

With the benefit of hindsight, I realise that I was a child who would worry about everyone else. I was sensitive to the words, actions and behaviours of others, and was easily overwhelmed by conflict and high emotion. As a child I recall sometimes feeling like I had a black cloud over my head. This would last for a few days, but always eventually passed. During these phases I wanted to be around people and sought comfort. I also recall having what I now understand to be panic attacks in response to a relationship breakup in my teenage years. I couldn't eat, wanted to isolate myself and felt lost.

Fast forward to my university years.

I loved university and developed a strong interest in psychiatry. The human psyche simultaneously fascinated and terrified me. With my empathetic and caring nature, I fell naturally into my therapy role. I was very driven and ambitious, so I chose to put myself into the most intense psychiatric environments you can ever encounter.

I worked in Broadmoor, a high security hospital with mentally ill offenders; in acute psychiatric wards with people experiencing a crisis in their mental health; in addictions and eating disorders, all the while being faced with the most dark and distressing stories I had ever heard. I tried my very best to put people back together again and gave it my all, often carrying the weight of the patient's distress on my shoulders.

I think I unknowingly took on too much at too young an age, with a fragile temperament. As a consequence of my own personality and experiences, coupled with the difficult situations I was facing every day, when I was twenty-five I developed my own story with anxiety.

A 'breakdown'; what does this look like? Is it a ranting moment when someone loses it and goes crazy, acting out of character? Is it a silent withdrawal, that person curled up into a ball and gently rocking? A place from where there is no return.

It is whatever your version looks like. I had a breakdown, but I didn't let myself 'break down'.

I had my first experience of diagnosable anxiety when, during a moment of high emotion and stress, I passed out in front of a group of patients. As you can imagine, this was hugely traumatic. I was completely blindsided. I felt out of control and terrified. This quickly escalated to a constant state of fear that this would happen again. I developed a fixation and fear of fainting, a phobia of that feeling of losing control.

I developed social anxiety which made it hard to stand in a queue in a shop, sit in a meeting, go out for a meal, or to generally be in a public place where people might see me. It began impacting on me to the point that I was filled with adrenaline all of the time - I couldn't eat or sleep. Even small tasks such as showering, getting ready to go out, planning or organising anything and phoning friends became too much for me.

I felt like the epitome of 'crazy'. Is this my breakdown? Will I end up in a locked ward? What if I lose everything?

I could not function. I could not live this terrifying life. I realised I needed help and went to my doctor. She prescribed me a low level of sertraline, an anti-depressant with an anxiolytic property, to help calm the feelings of anxiety I was experiencing. I understood that it would take a few weeks to start feeling the full effect of the medication, but I wasn't prepared for the immediate increase in symptoms.

I felt hyped up and agitated, my anxious and obsessional thoughts were louder, and it was even more difficult to sleep. Thankfully this calmed after the first week, and I began to see small improvements in my mental state.

Bit by bit I began to put myself together again. I frequently continued to experience flashes of adrenaline and panic, but I found that I was able to start to face things and live a little more of my life.

I would like to say that I'm now anxiety free, but the truth is that anxiety can still be my regular visitor. However, my whole mindset towards myself and my mental health has significantly altered. This is what has given me my life back.

Today I coach children, teens and adults to take care of their mental health. I deliver programmes in schools, talk at events and do individual therapy sessions with kids and parents who need a helping hand and a listening ear. I offer occupational therapy to transform mental wellbeing for the child and the supporting adult. My focus is on proactively nurturing good mental wellbeing using real-life, practical strategies so that clients can optimise on their potential and live a full life.

I have a professional and a 'lived experience' of mental health and its effects, and the service I provide reflects this. I can offer personal experience on what has worked, and I understand some of what a person is going through. It's therefore very authentic, and people warm to this quickly. I have a story to tell that has helped many, and I aim to gently guide an individual through their journey with kindness, compassion and humility. I regularly have feedback that I have helped people change their lives, and this is truly humbling.

Today I find myself training teachers, school staff and other businesses on the importance of self-care and proactive mental wellbeing. I do large presentations, trainings and public speaking events on average around six to eight times per month, and this is bearing in mind I have anxiety and previously would have avoided public speaking.

In the run up to a public speaking appointment, I am almost taken over by fear for the hour beforehand. I've come to accept that this is just part of what happens for me. I feel the fear, but I go on and do it anyway as this message is too important not to share.

Today my passion is to help others proactively look after their mental wellbeing by doing something every day that is good for them. To learn not to take their mental health for granted so that when crisis point hits, all hell breaks loose!

Can you see how I'm living my life despite my mental health challenges? You can, too.

Amidst my battle with my own mental health, I discovered a new self-awareness. An understanding of who I was. I realised that I was brave, that I had this strength and resilience I hadn't acknowledged before. I would not be the person I am now, and the entrepreneur making waves as I am, without having lived this experience.

When my mum died of breast cancer in 2011, I would have crumbled, had I not been through the darkness of my own mental health crisis a few years beforehand. I had the strategies, the self-awareness and the emotional understanding to realise that I could pull myself through whatever life launched at me.

Today, I really know who I am. I like myself. I respect and admire how I've coped with what I have, even though I often can't comprehend how I managed it. I have a personal understanding that whatever emotion I'm feeling will always settle and pass if I just let it. I might have a day when, for no apparent reason, I feel a little low or vulnerable, or higher in anxiety. I recognise now that this is okay, and that I won't always feel like this.

This is the message I want you to hear. To know that you can come back from 'rock bottom'. To know that every time you go through a relapse or setback, you develop a new understanding, a deeper sense of self and new strategies that will serve you going forward. To know that you can get through this, whatever this is for you, and come through the other side with a clearer under-standing of yourself. To know that where you are at just now does not mean you're always going to be here. To understand that right now you just need to hold on, for this moment will pass.

Why proactivity?

The World Health Organisation (2018) reports that *'mental health is a state of wellbeing in which an individual realises his or her own abilities, can cope with the normal stresses of life, can work productively and is able to make a contribution to his or her community.'*

The WHO states that society should act before a disorder such as depression is diagnosed and that it is not enough to acknowledge mental wellbeing at the point of diagnosis. Instead, *'proactive steps must be taken to promote and protect mental wellbeing throughout the life-span* (World Health Organisation, 2018).

Proactivity is essential. Imagine if we valued and treated our mental health like we do our physical health? On a daily basis, in order to keep ourselves physically well we may try to eat healthily, avoid excess alcohol and drink enough water. We know that physical exercise is good for us. We try to get enough sleep. We will tell people around us if we have a physical pain or ailment. We will happily visit a health professional for advice. We have no issue discussing this.

What about mental health? What steps do we consciously take to nurture good mental wellbeing on a daily basis?

Imagine if we didn't need to get to crisis point when everything starts to crumble. Imagine if I'd known how to keep myself well at a younger age? I think my adult life would have been on a completely different route. By proactively putting effort into mental wellbeing, on a daily basis as we do with our physical health, we can have a completely different experience. We can focus on 'mental wellbeing' as opposed to 'mental illness'.

Initially, in order to be proactive, I believe that we need to know and understand our own story and why we feel a certain way. Proactivity, for me, has been about learning to grow with or despite my anxiety. We can let awful situations affect us for evermore; colouring everything we do for the rest of our lives. Or we can choose to be brave, to start to open up and work through it.

We can acknowledge the pain and darkness, allow ourselves to grieve, feel the hurt, get angry and cry, with the knowledge that we can develop a deeper under-standing and move forwards, out of the pain. That over time the pain shifts and changes as you learn why you feel this way and what you can do to help yourself. At this stage, a great qualified practitioner will be able to help you find your way. Are you ready to do this?

Hand-in-hand with good self-awareness comes an under-standing of our triggers and boundaries, our preferences, dislikes and passions. We understand what motivates us and makes us tick. We begin to see what is important to us in life. When you know yourself in this way, you have a much better ability to handle life and all it throws at you.

Proactivity means, on a daily basis bringing to the forefront and habitually addressing our self-esteem, stress levels, self-talk, thoughts, emotions and mood - all of the core elements that keep us mentally well. We can do this by starting to practice strategies, find the ones that fit for us, then taking these on as a lifelong habit.

Proactivity promotes an openness and honesty about our mental wellbeing. One of the most vital steps we can take in our personal mental health journey, and as a society, is to start to talk about it. Instead of hiding behind "I'm fine", that we can start to express truly how we feel. So, if we feel stressed and anxious, we can say that. If our mood feels low and we are struggling with motivation, we talk about it. Can we start to do that? Can we start to normalise talking about the often hidden, more difficult emotions and mental health challenges?

I want to share some proactive methods of helping yourself with whatever it is that you are going through. Bear in mind that I've had many years of practice, and that you will need to pick out what you connect with and begin to develop it as a habit in your life. You might initially find some of the exercises difficult, but I ask that you don't give up and forget about them. Have a think, look at the questions, allow your mind to process. It might take you days, weeks or months to start to accep and apply some of this stuff, and I urge you to keep going because one day this will start to help if you let it.

Have faith that if you let it and if you apply the knowledge, this can really help you as it did me.

I also ask that you share this with your children, family, friends and colleagues because this will benefit them too. Even if they do not struggle with their mental wellbeing, by proactively nurturing the sense of self, we can all enjoy a more stable self-esteem, mood and level of stress.

Get yourself a lovely new notebook and practice engaging with yourself on a daily basis.

Your proactivity

This is your story and that's okay

Firstly, acknowledge that this is YOUR unique experience and story. You do not need to justify or explain it to anyone. This is happening to you and no-one else will ever appreciate how you feel. Lots of people will try to give you helpful advice, maybe tell you "to snap out of it," perhaps ask what you've got to feel anxious or depressed about. Disregard this - this is your story and you're going through this because you must. We don't always know the reason, but there often is something to be worked out or experienced.

What's your story? I realised quickly that I was putting

a box and labelling myself negatively. Why ne want to be with me, this crazy and anxious felt that people would only see my mental illness, not me, and this started to eat away at my confidence and self-belief. Let's get this straight - **you are so much more than that label**. Anxiety, depression, dyslexia, attention deficit hyperactivity disorder, autistic spectrum disorder, a physical health condition like multiple sclerosis, cerebral palsy, you have so much more to you.

Yes, I can be anxious and neurotic, but I'm also loving, gentle, smart, articulate and funny. I'm skilled at what I do. I have the ability to help someone shift towards a more positive mindset. I have a story to share, what about you?

Action

Start to note some of the other things about you. What are your strengths?

What are the challenges you've been through? What are your successes and achievements?

What are the positive things around your personality? If this is difficult, try to view it from another person's perspective. What would someone who really cares about you say?

What roles do you have in your life - mum, dad, carer,

friend, daughter, son, colleague, staff member? Write down the positive traits or skills someone with this role needs to be able to do a good job? Is this you?

What's great about your physical body, why do you appreciate it? What do you like about your appearance?

Continue adding to this list, without holding back, trying to give up on the 'if's or buts'. Write without concern for what others would think, write without restraint if you can. Try to let go just a little.

Give yourself credit for all of the things you are and do. I really believe that this is key in our mental health and wellbeing. This is not about ego or bragging. This is about healthy self-respect and a quiet self-belief, and this is what we need to nurture in order to aid a better mental wellbeing. When we are calm and confident in ourselves, when we know who we really are and come from a place of certainty, the actions and words of others, and the external events around us have less impact. Self-acceptance is vital to our mental wellbeing.

Your thoughts and words matter

What statements do you tell yourself on a day-to-day basis? "I'm a terrible Mum," "I'm fat and ugly and no-one likes me," "I can't do anything right," "I might as well give up". I've heard such statements from children right through to adults. How does this serve us?

Evidence demonstrates that thoughts impact on feelings,

and that this has a direct bearing on our behaviour and outcomes. So, if I'm saying to myself, "I'm useless. I can't do this; I don't have anything useful to contribute", what do you think I might feel like? Possibly low in self-esteem, angry, upset, anxious, sad. Then I might avoid that opportunity, I might self-isolate, I might fall out with my husband or shout at my kids. If this goes on long enough I might just reach that rock bottom. Can you see the pattern?

However, if I say to myself, "I can do this, I've done it before, I can do it again. I am doing just fine", how different might I feel? I'll feel encouraged, hopeful, a little more confident. My anxiety might be less.

Even in my darkest moments, I used mantras to help me hold on. "I believe in myself to get through this; this will pass, everything passes", became my stock phrase. What mantra can you use?

If only someone had taught me when I was a child that my thoughts are not always true, accurate, helpful or realistic. Sometimes they are based on childhood experiences and perceptions or false facts. We do not have to believe every thought that enters our head! We are not our thoughts and in fact, we can take a step back and choose not to engage.

Action

Take a moment now to write down any unhelpful or

negative statements you say to yourself. You might not realise that you are doing this, but just notice your thoughts, maybe even keep a thought diary for the next seven days and see what patterns come up.

You can then challenge the thought. If your thought is, "I fail at everything", start by finding all the evidence that backs this statement up. Show me the proof. Write down all of your examples.

Next, find all the evidence against this statement, that disproves the thought. So, in this situation, note all of the times that you haven't failed, your successes and achievements. You might find that there is more evidence against this unfair statement than for, and therefore begin to realise that this thought is false. What, therefore, is the more helpful and realistic statement? Your new statement might be, "I've achieved so much, and I can do this".

The words you say to yourself on a daily basis really matter. They have a massive impact on your self-esteem, mood, and mental wellbeing. You can be your own cheerleader.

You deserve to live your own best life

As adults, we often put ourselves last. Life takes over, we become busy with work, keeping house, raising a family, supporting others, and generally trying to keep afloat. We run through our days, juggling tasks, keeping everyone on track, racing from weekend to weekend, holiday to holiday.

We often lose ourselves just a little. We forget what lights us up and makes us feel excited. We let our goals slip, and neglect to do the things that make us feel happy. Before we know it, five, ten years have passed with us just 'living'.

But here's the thing - you really matter. Your happiness, hopes, dreams and goals count. You deserve to do the things in your life that you want to do, because this right here is it. This is your life.

Action

Take a moment now to think about all of the activities you've done before. What did you love to do? What have you put on hold?

What makes you happy now, what makes you feel good? What brings you a wholesome sense of calm? We do not need to make grand gestures or find hours of time for our happiness. Small things and quiet pauses each day really count. Lighting a candle, a hot cup of tea, deadheading flowers, drawing, singing, walking around the block. These all work for me.

From the things that make you feel happy and calm, could you find five or ten minutes every single day to do one of these? This might mean that you spend less time scrolling Facebook, get up slightly earlier, or take time before bed at night. Find that time, protect it, and start to do something every single day just for you and your wellbeing.

If you're in that place where everything seems too momentous, can you start at the very first step? Standing in the fresh air for a moment today, might tomorrow become a two-minute walk around the block. Put one foot forward and take the very next step, one foot in front of the other, until living starts to feel doable again. Today, get dressed; message a friend; get outside. Sometimes the very thing that we are avoiding is exactly what we need to do to start to find ourselves again.

When we take time out to nourish ourselves, we have more to give others. This type of self-care is not selfish; we need not feel guilty. It is indeed vital to our wellbeing and therefore has a knock-on effect to those around us, to our engagement with and productivity in society.

Just take the first step

> *"Take the first step in faith. You don't have to see the whole staircase, just take the first step"*
>
> **(Martin Luther King Jr).**

Following self-reflection comes action. What do you want to do first to start to work on your mental wellbeing? What area needs attention?

What is your commitment to yourself? Find the very first step, plan it and do it. Don't give up because it feels tough or is not working, keep going until it feels easier, until your confidence develops, and it becomes a good habit.

Proactivity means that you carry on doing the things that are good for your mental health and wellbeing habitually, daily and for the rest of your life. Because you know that they are good for you and keep you well. Because you're important and you matter; because life needs you to show up. Do not wait for crisis point - start now.

AUTHOR BIO

JILL TREVENA

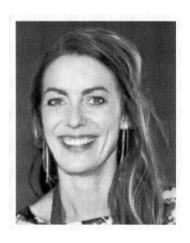

Jill Trevena is the founder of Practical Mindset.

She is a registered occupational therapist with twenty years' experience in assisting people to manage their mental and physical wellbeing and improving their quality of life.

Jill takes pride in offering the best therapy approach and providing 'gold standard' care. She provides a unique, creative and bespoke approach to mental health and wellbeing.

Jill's vision is to provide a person-centred mental health service that gets to the heart of the individual, their hopes, dreams and goals.

Jill aims to provide help in times of need. She is a strong voice in advocating proactivity in mental health and believes that by focusing on keeping a person mentally well, we are less likely to reach crisis point in mental illness.

Jill works in schools UK-wide, coaching children and their supporting adult, teacher, support staff or parent to learn and apply practical approaches to positive mental wellbeing. Sessions are outcome-focused, and the client is advised to use strategies consistently as part of their daily routine for maximum benefit.

Jill runs class sessions for pupils around core mental wellbeing topics including self-esteem, stress and anxiety, and emotions. She also runs sessions for children with additional support needs such as autistic spectrum disorder, attention deficit hyperactivity disorder and dyslexia.

Jill is the author of the Practical Mindset Toolkit for schools, a comprehensive mental health and wellbeing resource that is used to imbed mental wellbeing into the school curriculum.

Jill is regularly asked to present her work across Scotland.

Jill offers parent and child sessions to develop strategies for wherever the child is with their mental wellbeing, and additionally assists parents to find their way with the challenges they are facing.

Jill is also accomplished at running online programmes for kids, teens and parents.

Jill has her own story of mental health challenges and the service she provides reflects this. She can offer personal experience of what has worked for her, with an understanding of some of what a person is going through.

With her professional mental health experience, training and knowledge, she is equipped to work with people if they display signs of a more complex condition such as obsessional compulsive disorder or anxiety.

In addition to her mental wellbeing work, Jill carries out medico legal occupational therapy assessments and provides reports detailing care needs.

Jill has a story to tell that has helped many, and she aims to gently guide an individual through their journey with kindness, compassion and humility. She has received feedback that she has helped many people change their life, and she feels truly privileged to be a part of this journey.

Jill loves singing, snowboarding, yoga and holidays. She is an animal lover and her two dogs and rabbits are part of her family.

Jill is a committed gymnastics mummy, and a lover of life who wants others to experience their very best.

Follow and connect with Jill on Linkedin:

https://www.linkedin.com/in/jill-trevena-28818131

facebook.com/practicalmindsettherapy

twitter.com/trevena_jill

instagram.com/jill.trevena.practicalmindset

12

JOANNA BACON

hen do you decide something has to change? That you can't live your life consumed by depression any longer?

For me, it was a split-second moment.

I had suffered with high-functioning anxiety for years, which lead to depression and suicidal thoughts – Knowing what I know now, I presume it was down to a string of life-changing events, but most importantly – it was a lack of structure, discipline and healthy habits within my life.

I never realised, until I started to recover, just how important what I was doing on a daily basis, was. If you had told me 3 years ago that food, drink, sleep, exercise, thoughts and feelings all had an impact on my mental health, I would have laughed. I was always led to believe that mental health was caused by a chemical imbalance in your brain that you just couldn't help – it picked you, you didn't pick it.

Then I realised - everything that my life had become, everything that I was doing, everything that I was consuming both mentally and physically – caused the chemical imbalance.

My mental health problems started as a form of high functioning anxiety. For almost 2 years, I barely left the house, and if I did leave the house, it would take me anything up to 2 hours to actually leave my car to walk into my destination. I was fearful of everything, and everyone around me. That in itself, made me feel even worse. How do you explain to your partner that it took you 3 hours to do the food shopping, because you were too scared to get out of the car and walk into the shop?

I thought that not leaving the house would keep me safe, that it would make me feel better – but little did I realise, this was contributing to my poor mental health. You don't realise that when you're in the bubble of anxiety and depression, you think that it's easier/safer to stay at home – But once you start to go out into the world, you realise just how much life has passed you by, and the opportunities you've missed out on.

I lost friends because of poor mental health. In your head you want to be out having fun, spending time with your friends, making the effort to show up – But in reality, it's easier to say no and stay in your bubble of safety, or to pretend you're busy. If I did go and see my friends, I would be sat with my own thoughts telling myself, "Why am I here? No one likes me, do they? Why did they ask me to come? Surely, I should just leave? They would have so much more fun without me here, wouldn't they?", or I would distract myself by looking down at my phone.

My phone became my security anchor when out and hiding my anxiety. I would walk into a shop and pretend to be busy looking at my phone – So no one would approach me, talk to me, or notice my sadness and poor mental health. I'd do the same around my friends, family and partner – and little did I know, it didn't just stop them from seeing my poor mental health, it made them think I didn't value their time, presence and friendship.

Mental health consumed every reasonable thought I ever had. Every time someone I cared about left my side, I would fear for their life. "What if there is a car crash? What if my son gets taken? What if there's a terrorist attack? What if we get broken into? What if some attacks me?" – A million scenarios would go through my head on a daily basis.

If I watched anything negative on the media, I would have severe anxiety that I was next. I would avoid important phone calls, letters, emails – because in my head, there was a made-up scenario of everything going wrong once I answered them. It was easier to just say nothing, at all.

Enough became enough, after years of living like this. I remember the day like it was yesterday, that I was ready to ask for help. I was genuinely scared for my own life, and I knew I had to get help as soon as possible. I rang the doctors, to be told there was a 3 week wait, and that no one could see me. I broke.

I got off of the phone and rang a family member, with a background in the medical profession to ask for her advice, and thankfully within minutes I was booked in for the next day with her explaining the seriousness of my mental health. I worry now, how many people never make that 3 weeks wait?

The next few months saw me put onto the highest dosage of medication available for me. Thankfully, the anxiety started to ease, and my mind wasn't running at 100mph anymore.

And then I realised, my mind wasn't running at all. I slept most of my days away, I stopped getting up, I had no energy, I was fatigued, I was living pointlessly. I was living in a different world to the one I had been in, with my anxiety. Everything was slow, there were no thoughts, no feelings, I was just 'nothing'. I stopped going out, the washing piled up high, the house was a mess, I wasn't looking after myself, I lived in pyjamas, and hid my sadness behind a mask on social media.

And there it was, I'd swapped my severe anxiety, for severe depression.

I will never forget my turning point, that split-second moment I decided things had to change. I was in Sainsburys with my eldest son, waiting at a till, and as he spoke, my head turned to him, but my eyes didn't. I was so spaced out, I didn't know what planet I was on. It was like I was living in a bubble with no feelings, and no existence.

That split second, is where things changed. That split second, is where I realised – nothing was ever going to be 'OK' until I took control of this illness myself. Taking medication was masking the problem, not dealing with it, and taking the medication only ever gave me more side effects, and less feelings.

I reached out to a close friend. We'd been through similar life changes and had been helping each other through the hard times. I noticed he was starting to evolve through the darkness, and I wanted some advice on how. His advice was simple, he told me to order a programme which would help to re-programme my brain and give me natural serotonin and dopamine releases (everything my medication was doing, without the side effects). I didn't question it, I just ordered it.

One day. One day, is all it took to notice a difference. Of course, I wasn't cured from mental health within one day, but there was light at the end of a very long, dark tunnel.

The programme consisted of two very important components. A book, which helped to re-programme my thinking, and a superfood shot, which contains Bioperine and Lions Mane Mushroom (scientifically proven to help raise serotonin and dopamine – naturally!).

As I looked at the book, I realised how simple the steps were, but how easy it was to overlook them. 7 simple steps, every single morning, taking no longer than 20 minutes to complete.

Who would have thought that if I didn't allow natural sunlight onto my skin first thing in the morning, I would affect my circadian rhythm, which in turn affects my hormone release, sleep cycles, eating habits and digestion, and more?

So, there was my first task. No more snoozing the alarm, no more laying in bed scrolling through social media with the curtains closed. Straight away, as soon as I woke up, I had to be up and in natural sunlight.

The simplest task, yet one that many of us would never deem as important, until we see the true benefit ourselves.

The second task, came as even more of a shock to me, when I read the studies behind it. Drink water within the first 20 minutes of the day? If I was being honest with myself, I was barely drinking water at all, I was living on caffeine to get me through the tired days. Little did I know then, that it was contributing to my poor mental health.

I did a study with a group of clients a few months ago, to see how many people were dehydrated, and also checked in on their mood levels – and what did I find? The people that drunk more water, had a higher 'happiness score', than those who didn't make it a priority.

Even being mildly dehydrated can impact your mood, reduce your motor and cognitive function, affect your memory and energy levels. So, there it was, my second task, to ensure I had a litre of water within the first 20 minutes of my day, to nourish my body and set it up for the day. And what do you know? It started to help.

The third task, was my biggest fear – movement! I thought when I read movement, that I would be going from sleeping all day, to running 5K every day! But again, it was simple, it was doable, it was achievable. Did you know that alongside the blast of light on your skin in the morning, getting up and moving straight away wakes your body up and again, sets your circadian rhythm?

There was me thinking I would have to be running miles to feel better and get 'happy hormone' releases – but it was as simple as getting straight up, walking downstairs, drinking my litre of water, whilst running around the house after my crazy toddler! The difference from laying in bed snoozing next to my toddler watching TV, was huge.

And that's one of the biggest things that has come from my recovery, and completion of this programme daily – The effect it has had on my children. From creating good habits, myself, I have instilled good habits into them. I now regularly practice gratitude and reflection with them and setting tasks – as I know how much of a huge impact it had on my life, and mental wellbeing.

After getting natural light on my skin, moving around, and drinking a litre of water – then came the secret potion. Every single day I had to take a superfood blend consisting of 36 of the most powerful superfoods from around the world. This wasn't any old superfood I could buy in a store, it was an award-winning blend of vitamins, minerals and antioxidants. Each ingredient was scientifically selected and cultivated for its powerful health benefits, given in the shot at clinical dosages to ensure it had positive effects on the body.

I only had to research two of the 36 ingredients, to understand how they helped me – Lions Mane Mushroom, and Bioperine – proven to help anxiety, depression, raise serotonin and dopamine, improve memory and brain function. It was no coincidence that I was healing.

All of these things were powerful – but the real work came when I had to complete a daily journal. When I first looked at the journal, I couldn't see how it could possibly help me to feel better – but of course, you don't realise until you do, just how much little steps in the right direction, take you to the right path.

Every single day I was to journal three things I was grateful for. Sure, we all say it in our heads, but there is a huge impact once you start to write it down. Gratitude works because it slowly changes the way we perceive situations by adjusting what we focus on, it overpowers negative emotions. If we focus on all the bad, everything will feel bad. If we focus on the good there is in our life, our energy is focused on the good. Remember, where focus goes – energy flows.

The idea is to change what you're grateful for every day, so that your mind starts to expand to the good that is in your life. Of course, if you're in a bad place mentally, it can make you feel that there is no good in the world – but once you start to open your eyes and mind to gratitude and finding something good in the world, everything changes.

Next, I was to set myself three tasks to complete every single day. Again, you wouldn't understand the power of this, until you start to do it.

Let's be honest, when you're in a bad place, the last thing you think about is setting a goal for the day. Because you have so much to do. I know when I was in the height of my anxiety and depression – nothing got done, which made me feel even worse.

The house was a mess, the dishwasher was never done, the washing was piled up until we had no clothes to wear and I HAD to do some washing, the food shop was always last minute, we ate too many takeaways, my business wasn't given enough attention, my accounts were never done, I wasn't replying to texts/calls/emails. There were so many bad habits. But it was time to tackle them one by one.

In the early days my tasks were simple – Get a load of washing done, empty and fill the dishwasher, and cook a healthy meal for my family. You don't realise at first, but once you write those tasks down, your mind will continue to remind you throughout the day, that the tasks need to be done – and you do them!

What's even better, is when you complete a task, your body will have a rush of dopamine – a happy hormone. We live in a generation whereby people live for 'likes' on social media, and their dopamine releases are from a fake reality. This is an incredible way to ensure you're getting natural dopamine releases. The more tasks you complete, the happier you will feel, as you start to feel your life is getting back on track.

Once you start to complete tasks every single day, over a period of time, they become a habit. Now that I have been using this programme for over a year, I don't even think of the dishwasher, washing, or cooking as a task – it's a daily habit, its engrained into my life.

It was only once I started to work on the small, daily things, that I could set bigger tasks – things I had been putting off during the depth of my illness. It can feel overwhelming when you write a list of 30 things you need to do and have lacked doing whilst being ill – and it can feel like they'll never get done – But by breaking those 30 things, into 3 a day – Everything that has been avoided for weeks/months/years can be completed within 10 days.

This is how I got my life back on track, starting with smaller tasks, the essentials, making them a habit, and then moving onto the things that were really going to get me to where I wanted to be in life – my big goals!

Every 15 days during my programme I would have to chart my happiness scores – I would look at my overall mood, gratitude, hydration, sunlight, movement, health, execution of tasks, mindset and energy levels. The increase, within the first 56 days, was astonishing.

So, was I magically healed after one day, week, or month on this programme? The answer is no.

Bad mental health cannot be healed overnight, or over weeks, or months. Mental health is something you wake up to every single day of your life and face head on, it's a battle you choose to face, and win.

My mental health is controlled by habits – If I practice good habits, using the programme – I am well. If I start to practice bad habits and ignore the simple steps I have to take every morning and day, my mental health goes downhill. It's an everyday fight. I realised that my reality is only ever as good as my habits.

I noticed within a very short space of time of starting to change my daily habits, that my weeks went from having six bad days and one good day, to six good days, and only one bad. The bad days got less, and when the bad days came – I knew how to deal with them better.

Within just six weeks, I had taken myself off of the incredibly high dosage of antidepressants I was on, that were causing horrific side effects, and I was managing my mental health by simply following the simple steps in the programme, and drinking my superfood shot every single day.

Six months after starting the programme, my real test came.

I was pregnant with twins, and I went for a private scan to see my babies. I was told that one of my babies' heart had stopped beating, but that the other was growing fine.

As you can imagine, like any mother in this situation, I didn't know how to think or feel. I had to wait another week for a second scan, to check that my second baby was OK, only to have my heart shattered and be told that both of them had died inside the womb.

Within 24 hours, both of my babies were taken from my

body, and taken to be tested on, and then cremated. Within 24 hours, my entire world had changed.

I felt numb, but I knew one very important thing – my mental health was a priority, and during this time, I would either sink or swim. I knew myself well, and I knew that I could hit rock bottom with a click of a finger – or I could stand up and fight.

I allowed myself time to be numb, to cry, and to grieve. I took time away from my business and created a little hobby to keep myself busy. But most importantly, I started back on my mindset programme. I practiced gratitude every single day. Of course, at a time like this, what was there to be happy about? But when I looked around, there was a lot to be happy about – my beautiful children, my home, my family. I set myself small tasks again, to get me back on my feet – they were simple, but they kept me focused.

Six weeks after the loss, everything hit me like a tonne of bricks. I was grieving, I was hormonal, and there were problems within my relationship. I was due to meet a friend in London, and I didn't know whether I could face it – But I knew that if I went, I would feel better for going. I cried the whole way there, and when I got to the London underground, my emotions became so overwhelming, I questioned my life.

I looked at the train approaching the platform at speed, and I was seconds away from throwing myself in front of it. I didn't think about how it might affect my family, my children – I didn't want to die, but I just wanted the pain to end. I remembered everything I had been taught from my programme, and I forced myself to sit down.

Believe me when I say, it was so hard to sit down, that I had to physically hold the rails to stop myself from getting up and ending my life. I composed myself and I retrained my thoughts. In the split second I was about to end my life, I retrained my thoughts. I always wonder if an angel was sent down to me that day.

Not one person around me noticed me, not one person said a thing.... But one man, came and stood in front of me and blocked my path to the platform. Was it deliberate? I'll never know. Was it an angel sent? I'll never know. All I know, is that day I got a second chance at life.

If thinking of three things I am grateful for, would raise my happiness levels by 10%, would that 10% be enough to pull me from suicidal, to life?

It worked. It actually worked.

I missed two trains, as I composed myself, but as I got onto the third train, in a wave of relief, fear and gratitude – I questioned. How many people didn't stop themselves? How many people couldn't stop themselves in that very moment? I went on to have a lovely day with my friend, and go home as normal, how many people don't get that second chance?

The answer is over 5000 people per year.

It was from that day, I made it my life's mission to ensure that everybody knew my story, and knew that there was something, an alternative option in the world, that may help them to live a fulfilling life, and not rely on medication.

It was from that day that I dedicated my time to help people who suffer from anxiety and depression, and give them a safe place to talk, network, and connect.

My life isn't perfect, and there are still good and bad days, however – with the knowledge I have, of understanding how my brain works, and how I can naturally raise my hormone levels – I battle those bad days head on. I still, to this day, years on from the battles of anxiety and depression, practice everything I did then, because I know that the mind is the most powerful thing we own. If the mind is the most powerful thing we own, then we must work on it daily.

I share my story in the hope that it will help someone else see that there is light at the end of every tunnel.

JOANNA BACON

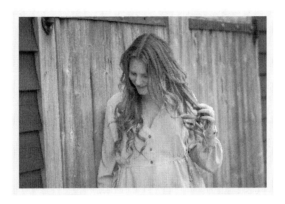

Joanna Bacon is an extremely successful business women, running multiple businesses all over the world. After becoming a mum at 16 she strived to create success for her family and graduated 5 years later with a degree in Business Management.

She used this Business Management Degree to build her multiple businesses resulting in tcams of thousands of people all over the world, also building flexible businesses from home. She specialises in health and wellness, travel and money management.

This career move has allowed Joanna to be a stay at home

mum, expand her family and take multiple trips around the world each year, as well as winning multiple awards for top performance in her companies.

As well as her networking businesses, she is also a Self-Love and Mindset Coach, and a Business Coach teaching people to succeed through their struggles. She runs a Self-Love and Mindset Community aimed at women looking to work on themselves after suffering Anxiety and Depression, or Trauma in their lives.

Joanna's vision is to positively impact as many lives as possible in her time – however that may be!

Contact:

joannaleyanbacon@hotmail.com

Facebook -

https://www.facebook.com/joannabaconglobal/

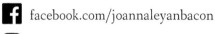 facebook.com/joannaleyanbacon

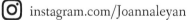 instagram.com/Joannaleyan

13

PAULINE LAWSON

"You can't start the next chapter of your life if you keep re-reading the last one"

Tiny Buddha - Unknown

a few years ago my own mental health took a bit of a hit. I suffered panic attacks, frequent overwhelm, sleeplessness, and lack of energy.

I could sit here, catastrophise, and focus on a huge list of negatives, however as a 'future focussed' person I choose not to. Due to my personal journey in self-development I prefer to think about it for what it is; a piece of my past, a learning experience, and a stepping stone to my next chapters.

I look back upon this now with gratitude.

It is hard to pinpoint a time when I wasn't able to reframe events and situations habitually, and to look upon challenging times with this more grateful, positive, and accepting outlook. What I do know is that if anyone had mentioned 'gratitude' or 'being grateful' during the darker moments, I may have thrown a gratitude journal at them! I will often tell those that I support in my work, life is not all glitter and unicorns, nor would we want it to be. Life is real and we have to put in a little bit of work to find and create our own glitter!

I now notice if my mental health is slipping and take appropriate action. Knowing this is all part of my being resilient.

Looking back I can recall that this period of my life was filled with signs, messages, critical incidents and catalyst moments. I was eventually forced to listen to all of these messages.

With the help of friends, loved ones, and professionals, I worked out that I had 'Work Related Stress'. There it was, the working area of my life was damaging my health.

I took a while, but I made a decision to leave behind a huge part of my life and what I thought, at the time, was a big part of my identity - my career within education.

I took the leap, but something within me decided not to be scared. I chose to be excited.

I knew I wasn't going off to do nothing, as that is not really my style. I put my energy and creativity into doing exactly the same as I had been doing for many years. Supporting and educating children, young people, their families, and wider professionals to work on their Emotional Literacy, Mental Health, and Emotional Wellbeing proactively, to have the skills in place to deal with adversity in more healthy ways.

No Rose-tinted Glasses or Catastrophising

I look back now and actively choose to see the fortunate parts within my career.

I worked as a teacher, spent time in different roles as a Principal Teacher, and eventually as a Deputy Head. For most of my career I was working with children, young people, and families living with huge adversity, with these adversities impacting on their day-to-day school lives.

I had the privilege of taking my career in a direction where I was able to support young people, and those around them, in learning to work with mental health in healthier ways.

However I don't wear rose-tinted glasses. My work held its challenges and not always in the places many people believed the challenges to be.

My saddest times were when I felt like a square peg in a round hole; feelings of loneliness, even amongst a sea of colleagues. Times when I struggled to find more than a handful of like-minded thinkers, a sense of belonging. Not always able to move things forward as was needed and having to watch young people, who were already facing adversity, face even more.

At times it all seemed more than my head and heart could cope with. But each time I picked myself up, and tried again, and again, and again.

What was happening around me at the lowest times began to bring up feelings of doubt and shame within me for doing what I do, being who I am. Living in line with our values makes us who we are and my values were being challenged daily.

Something changed, internally or externally, or maybe a combination of both. Something made me stop and take a step back and I realised the waves were coming too thick and fast and my voice was becoming lost in the wind.

I wasn't helping **me**. My cup was empty, and therefore I wasn't helping my children and young people.

I am proud that I went on to use my time and creativity as a business owner to build up my training, skills, and business, carrying myself forward into the world beyond education. I am now a Transformational Life Coach, and Emotional Wellbeing and Mindfulness Coach, and I continue to develop and use creative approaches to work alongside all people, to support them to add value to their own lives.

Myth Busting

I also feel it is important to say that I work with kids who very often have an overflow of emotion led by their life circumstances. This can often be displayed in loud, rude, aggressive, and even violent ways.

I hear phrases like this,

"Ohh, did you give up teaching because of the kids? I know you worked with the tough ones",

or even,

"I'm not surprised that you gave up, some of these kids nowadays, they need stronger discipline",

and wait for it,

"Teachers have no power anymore, we should bring back the belt".

These are the ones that I can actually write down!

My answer to all of these is **no!** My kids were not the reason I felt I had to move on from formal education. The kids were my reason for keeping on going. These kids have been some of my best teachers.

"She stood in the storm and when the wind did not blow her way, she adjusted her sails."

Elizabeth Edwards

What is Resilience?

I recall a catalyst incident that happened within my workplace when I was in a tough spot with my mental health. I will share, not for the purposes of drama but because these memorable moments often hold the biggest lessons.

The conversation goes along these lines, all said in quite a matter of fact way,

"I thought you were more resilient than this, Pauline",

My heart missed a couple of beats. I thought my emotional brain may kick in and someone may need to pass me the tissues, but no, my thinking brain, and almost certainly my training and experience, stepped up.

I was then able to reply...

"Oh I am very resilient, I just believe we have two very different versions of what resilience really means"

Short and not so sweet, but this left me with a strange mix of clarity and puzzlement around the range of different ways resilience is defined.

· · ·

Language is Important

The more I thought about this conversation my solution-seeking mind was running different little 'resilience' movies I have lived and seen over and over.

I had studied resilience factors and taught resilience skills to kids and families that live with ongoing adversity in their lives. I felt I had a pretty good idea of what resilience looked like and felt like in real life.

I believe with all my knowledge and heart that a huge part of resilience is listening to your emotions and feelings and working 'with' these. Not hiding them away and just taking on the 'Dig Deep', 'Carry on Regardless', 'More Effort' approaches.

Reaching out, seeking support and solutions, showing vulnerability, leaning in on the supports and skills you have available. To me, these are all acts of strength and courage, and necessary parts of being resilient.

This was probably the time when it hit me that there were many, many different interpretations of the word 'resilience'. With many interpretations of resilience in existence, this means people are, at times, speaking a different language to one another. Therein lies a danger zone. Language is so important that a lack of clarity or mismatch can cause uncertainty and therefore cause mistakes and create fear.

Resilience isn't a Fixed Trait

There is amazing research around the whole range of skills that a person can benefit from having in place, to hold a higher level of resilience. Sounds like a simple concept, and absolutely one I hold onto within my work.

My preferred understanding of resilience comes from research and is also continually inspired by my lived experiences. It has always been about placing a focus on learning, building, and maintaining a range of positive life skills and habits. The layering up of these gives us strong foundations, creating a compound effect, and allows us all to hold an optimum level of resilience in any given situation.

Development of **skills**, giving **strong foundations**, and layering up, creates **resilience.**

Tried & Tested

'Leaning In'

Part of my own survival toolkit during periods when my mental health is at its lowest, is remembering that whilst one part of my life is dipping I have other areas within my life that are full, secure, and safe. When my work life dipped I was able to use these other areas to provide a scaffold, to call upon for strength, support, and maintain some sort of balance.

This is something I refer to as 'Leaning In'.

)f Life' coaching approach, a person can
:as of their life and create a visual repre-
is. To do this, use a big circle sliced up like
each segment labelled to represent an area
ot y~   , e.g. family, work, relationships, social life,
health, exercise, diet, fun & leisure, finance. These pizza
slices can be shaded in or numbered on a scale of 1-10,
with 10 being all going really well and 1 really not going
so well. Creating a Wheel of Life visual allows people to
identify the areas that are causing the discomfort and
also the stronger areas, and these are where the 'Leaning
In' strategy can take place.

Having these strong areas within our lives truly provides
the resilience that we can tap into when needed. Even
when one part of our life is dipping, this does not necessarily mean any of us are falling or failing. It certainly
does not mean we need to accept any labels as a Non-
Resilient Person.

For a period of time in my life, **me**, the teacher had to
become the learner. 'Leaning In' to the many areas of my
life that were strong and solid gave me breathing space
and feelings of safety, which enabled me to create my
own next steps.

We all need to remember that bank of resilience skills
that we have all held inside ourselves since we were little.
We all managed to pick ourselves up when learning to
walk, talk, eat – and algebra! We shouldn't worry if we

feel our resilience banks are a little low, as resilience skills **can** also be strengthened and learnt, and we can all use a bit of 'Leaning In' when needed.

What I have found successful for developing skills in resilience, is to remember those areas of our life that are going well, maybe something sitting higher on the Wheel of Life mentioned earlier. Our mind is much more open to practice a new skill within areas of our lives where there are less barriers or hurdles.

I have found it a hard sell to ask others, or even myself, to be grateful or look for positive aspects within an area of life which is sitting pretty low on The Wheel. Our brains have a natural negativity bias and it takes a lot more energy to create a habit of seeking positives.

The good news is that we all have the power to choose one thought over another and we do not have to 'hang out' with our low feelings. The momentum can be started by using the 'Leaning In' strategy; developing skills within an area that scored higher on The Wheel. Once a positive habit is formed, and within our brain a strong neural pathway has been created, then we can then set about applying this positive habit into an area of our lives that scored lower on The Wheel.

A personal example of this is when I found it a real challenge to develop a gratitude habit within my work life while it was very scoring low on my Wheel. I used the higher scoring areas of family and friends to develop a gratitude habit within those areas and it was then easier to find the positives. Having a strong positive habit and therefore building a strong neural pathway, I could then transfer these skills and be able to look at my work life with a more positive mindset.

My work with people is always around building creative and pro-active strategies for strengthening the resilience muscle, and working on this every single day. This helps them to become 'life ready' for whatever comes next.

Me teaching the kids or the kids teaching me?

"It is important to remember that we all have magic inside us"

JK Rowling

A story of true resilience.

I worked with an amazing young lady who had lived with adversity since a very young age, with this ongoing adversity rippling into many areas of her life.

She had worked out that logically speaking there were lots of positive things around and about her that were true. But the heartbreaking thing for me was that she openly said, "I just don't like, love, or believe in me". She couldn't see or feel her own magic.

That was her moment. She was being open and vulnerable. She, like many others I support, didn't need my tears and my emotions thrown into the mix at that moment. I had to wear my big girl pants, and with a deep breath and not a bit of 'emotional leakage', I said to her, "Well don't worry too much about that for now. I will believe in you enough for both of us until you are ready to do it for yourself".

Following on from this we had many learning conversations following this up. She would check in to see if I still had this bag of self-belief for her. Sometimes we joked that it was getting heavy as we shared factual achievements and growth. She came to see if was I getting too old to carry it any longer. All of this... right up until a lovely moment came where she approached me and told me quietly that she felt ready to take it for herself. I will admit to a sneaky tearful moment then – but not too much. Just a ceremonial passing over of the 'bag'!

Many others believed and stated that this was a young lady with no resilience or staying power. I believe this learning process we went through together showed so many skills in resilience. Opening up and being vulnerable, searching out a key and trusted person to share this with and gain support, recognising her successes, and identifying the part that needed work.

We didn't 'hang out' with that low area within her life. She 'Leaned In' on the other areas of her life that were going well and built herself up. The layering of positive habits led to her having the strength to take charge of the self-belief.

Creative Approaches

> *"The Mental Health of our children must be seen as every bit as important as their physical health"*

HRH The Duchess of Cambridge

This quote resonates so much with me, as it has long been my mission to ensure that everyone has the opportunity to learn about their own mental health.

I would however like to exchange the word *children* within the quote for *nation*, as we do **all** have mental health. We can all experience good mental health and all experience poor or low mental health.

This is why we need to continually have our resilience foundations, skills, and positive habits in place, so that we are ready and able to look after our own mental health.

Learning and teaching around physical health is common, with advice on food, exercise, and hygiene all easily accessed. When the time is right we also learn and teach about sexual health, drugs, alcohol, and a range of other things that are good for us and bad for us. We learn too about keeping ourselves safe, and basic risk assessment, from a young age. We are then able to make sound choices around our own wellbeing.

I believe it is only reasonable that we all have the opportunity to learn and teach about all humans as 'emotional beings' and the responsibility we all hold in looking after our own and others mental health.

There are so many ways now of accessing and sharing robust knowledge, and having knowledge that we can put into action is powerful. Professionals have discovered so much about the brain and how it all works with regard to emotions and responses.

There are also life stories that can be shared, in person, in books, and social media, which can create a connectedness and a sense of belonging. Knowing that you are not alone in any given situation can be a huge boost to resilience.

As with any area of our health the phrase Mental Health encapsulates many things, and this often opens up controversy as to who can and cannot support this.

I, for one, am happy to play a part in preparing the current and next generation, as well as myself, in having some tools to enable and empower us to look after mental health, including knowing how to reach out if additional support is needed.

This is all part of having a strong Resilience Toolkit.

"Alone we can do so little, together we can do so much"

Helen Keller

As well as being a teacher, I am also a mum, partner, daughter, sister, auntie, cousin, niece, friend, colleague, life coach – and much more.

I teach because 'I am' not because I am 'a teacher'.

Connection and relationships are key to teaching; therefore, it is a job many of us can play a part in.

There isn't a workbook or full curriculum to teach about mental health, so I use the tools I have – my life skills, my compassionate approach, my unconditional positive regard for all, my tenacity... and a whole range of creative approaches that many others can adopt and adapt.

Here I will share ideas and concepts from my own experience that have been tried and tested on those aged 5-18 and adult coaching clients too.

Some classic self-development themes are embedded within these simple creative activities. One day I will write all of my creative ideas down to share.

"When you change the way you look at things, the things you look at change"

Wayne Dyer

Reframing

Reframing is a simple technique used in a range of therapies to support looking at things with a different perspective.

Kids love real picture frames for learning how to 'Reframe'.

It does somehow help to physically write down some of our big catastrophising thoughts around a situation that is causing anxieties, stresses, and fear. This is where the big frame comes in (a real frame or draw a big picture frame) and we give ourselves permission to get every thought written down within the frame.

Our minds can get pretty creative and with our brains having a natural negativity bias a wealth of unlikely scenarios may come up about a situation, almost like a mini disaster movie appearing in our minds. Fear engages the emotional part of our brain, and the logical and thinking part becomes disengaged.

Firstly, making changes to some emotive language can really help our minds feel calmer. Are you terrified or just a bit scared? Are you angry or are you irritated? Do you really hate that person or did you dislike the thing they did? We can then write some of the new less emotive language into our frame, rubbing out the emotive ones.

We can also challenge some of the unlikely scenarios. Is

your friend **never** going to speak to you again? Are you actually going to **lose** your job? Is **everyone** going to stare and laugh? This is a great process to work though, working back to the true situation and to an emotional state that allows us to think more logically.

We are learning that we have the power to change the movie and work out which thoughts are real, possible, likely, and unlikely. The reframing teaches the mind about the power of choice.

With the emotional part of the brain now soothed, the thinking part comes into play, helping us to come up with better solutions to something that a short while ago seemed just too big and overwhelming.

The new frame can now be filled with scenarios and situations that our brain **can** cope with. This may still be something troubling that needs to be addressed, but now we are in the correct mindset and have soothed our brain by changing the energy levels held within the frame.

These are the foundations for creating a simple reframing skill and habit that becomes one of our Resilience Skills to call upon when needed.

Rainbow Glasses

Gratitude is a hard gig to sell to anyone that is currently sitting with a negative mindset. What we do know is that having a healthy gratitude habit trains our brains, creating neural pathways inside it that allow us to seek and see positivity more clearly, even within difficult circumstances.

My Rainbow Glasses bring a little smile and humour to the hard work that has to be put into developing a healthy gratitude habit. Little kids, big kids, and even grown-ups, all love wearing the Rainbow Glasses.

Yes, I do have real glasses decorated with rainbows. I also have Grumpy Glasses, and other glasses decorated to represent a range of other moods such as anger, hate, nervousness, and excitement.

Kids have chosen or been tasked with wearing mood glasses all day to allow the experience and assessment of how it feels to be looking at the world with a certain outlook. When tried multiple times this opens up a dialogue of comparing and considering if one pair is preferable to another. This shows the kids that they do have the power of choice with which of their 'glasses' to wear and that focusing our energies on a specific mood can change our outlook.

Some examples have been with kids not feeling capable in a certain school subject, or hating the cinema because their sister chose the movie. The concept of Rainbow Glasses has been tried and tested with simple results such as focusing on the sums that were correct rather than those that were wrong; recalling the support from peers and teachers and how it helped; and to something as simple as focusing on enjoying the snacks at the cinema, finding enjoyable parts of the movie and remembering that it is their turn to choose the movie next time. It is not all about making life easy and pleasant with no hurdles, but about being able to set our minds to a more positive outlook.

Kids are often more motivated knowing that they have the power of choice. None of us like to be told to be a certain way or feel a certain feeling at any given time. It is empowering to know that we can choose to select the Rainbow Glasses if we feel ourselves dipping into a mood that is not helpful or too big.

All of this can lead kids to seeking and seeing more of the 'Rainbow Moments', instead of actively seeking the 'Darker Side' of any given day or situation. The more they choose the Rainbow Glasses (physically or metaphorically) then the more they develop a natural gratitude habit, and another resilience skill develops.

Foundations and Scaffolds

Kids can have worries around knowing if they are resilient or not. Placing themselves simply in one camp or another. The word needs a bit of unpicking and exploring for them.

It often helps kids to see resilience as a physical structure. I use pictures of The Eiffel Tower, The Leaning Tower of Pisa, and or even the ruins of a castle as visuals.

Kids see The Eiffel Tower as tall and straight, the Leaning Tower of Pisa as a little lopsided, and castle ruins as a bit tumbled. What they all have in common though is that they are still standing. Why? Because they have strong foundations and because some builders placed scaffolds in when needed. Kids know straight away that the tops of these towers and buildings would not be standing without the foundations.

On those pictures, or models built with construction materials, I work with kids to label the foundations with all the skills in their own lives that they believe are strong and are their own foundations. Kids do love to build and when their playful brain is engaged the flow comes into the dialogue. All the positive parts of their life are spoken about, all holding together to create a strong structure, a physical representation of the resilience they already hold. The Leaning Tower of Pisa image often comes up in discussions as a representation of not having to be perfect, but it is still standing!

The fact is that, on occasion, a building needs a bit of scaffolding to hold it up. Sometimes we need this too. Kids often feel the need to revisit their building when there are changes in their lives. They may feel they have lost a skill or not yet have a specific skill in place. In the same way as in the story where I held the bag of self-belief for one of my pupils for a short while, something or someone needs to hold the space within these kid's buildings until they are ready to do it themselves.

This is where the concept of 'Leaning In' comes in, as kids choose a 'scaffold' within their lives to hold that space. This could be a significant person or a different skill they currently feel confident in.

It doesn't really matter what or who. What matters is the space is being held, and their building (and therefore their resilience) will not fall down. This scaffold or space-holding is just long enough until they build up their own skills to fill the space.

The important thing here is that all of us need to know that we are not alone when we are hurting or our resilience is dipping. We need to reach out to people that will sit with us and scaffold us.

Through this learning resilience becomes further understood as a 'live' process that requires ongoing maintenance and looking after.

* * *

If you take one thing away from this chapter, I hope it is that resilience is about having a range of pro-active skills that you can dip into when your mental health is low. These skills will be your resilience toolkit that will help you through situations as they arise. If we hold onto that knowledge we can also share this with others.

Resilience isn't that 'one fixed thing'. It is something we can all take steps to continually build on and maintain throughout our lives. Resilience is a journey not a destination.

> *"Joy, collected over time, fuels resilience – ensuring we'll have reservoirs of emotional strength when the hard things happen."*

Brene Brown

AUTHOR BIO

PAULINE LAWSON

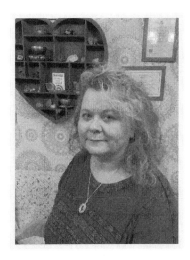

Pauline lives in Bonnyrigg near Edinburgh, Scotland with her long-term partner Keith and their grown-up son Danny. She has lived in this area for 20 years. Originally she is from Aberdeen in Scotland, which is where she spent most of her childhood years.

After studying and training for 5 years to gain a Bachelor of Education, Honours Degree, Pauline has had a 20 year career within Education, working as a Teacher,

Principal Teacher, and eventually a Depute Head Teacher.

Most of her education career has been working in and taking on leadership roles within schools and services that support children, young people, and families living with the impact of adversity.

Many of Pauline's roles have been based on adjusting the mindset and culture within schools and services to facilitate change and the implementation and use of more positive, supportive, and compassionate discipline approaches, which support emotions and therefore behaviours.

Pauline has been on a self-development journey of her own, for many years, to support her own mental health issues and has gone on to study a whole range of holistic and therapeutic approaches. These include Reiki, Emotional Freedom Technique, CBT Approaches, NLP approaches, Aromatherapy, Indian Head Massage and Mindfulness.

She is also qualified as a Youth Mindfulness Coach for Kids and Teens, Relax Kids Coach, Story Massage Facilitator, Positivity Practitioner, and a Transformational Life Coach.

Pauline has used this training and experience to create and build her own business called ***EmotionAll Coaching and Emotional Wellbeing Services.***

In the time that Pauline has had her own business she has hosted regular local child and teen classes and one-to-one sessions to support all in learning more about emotions and wellbeing.

Using a blend of creative approaches, she empowers and supports others to look after their emotions in the healthiest of ways. Alongside this she continues to be invited to work within education for a range of purposes. This includes working alongside amazing schools, teachers, and children, to support the development of key parts of the Health and Wellbeing Curriculum.

In many schools she provides consultations and development opportunities for schools and staff to learn practical skills to support their own mental health and enable them to more fully support the children they work with. There are also opportunities for working with parents to support a shared message around wellbeing, therefore making a bigger impact on our children and young people. Support and sessions also continue for local associations such as local youth football clubs, after school clubs, and Brownies.

Pauline also offers Transformational and Empowerment Life Coaching to teens and adults, both face-to-face and online. To reach a wider audience her next steps will be to create and facilitate more coaching groups for children, teens, and adults.

In amongst all of this Pauline ensures she doesn't let time

for leisure and hobbies slide. One of her favourite ways to switch off, have thinking space, and some fun is to have trips away with Keith in their motorhome. Frequently touring far and wide in Scotland and the UK, making use of the amazing scenery and walking opportunities.

Whilst travelling and touring Pauline makes the most of this time and writes blog posts, sharing all her thoughts and experiences across the world of education, self-development, and coaching.

Pauline also enjoys yoga, Pilates, and fitness classes and continues to improve her practice in all of these, keeping up with a 'healthy body, healthy mind' approach.

She also enjoys making and creating things, cards, jewellery, home decorating, and experimenting with other creative endeavours. The creation of various crafts also finds its way into support sessions with children and teens.

As Pauline continues to learn and share more in the world of self-development and transformational life coaching she ensures that she continues to create a life fully in line with her values.

Pauline can be contacted currently on Social Media :-

Wordpress

https://emotionallthings.wordpress.com

Linkedin

https://www.linkedin.com/in/paulinelawson-EmotionAll/

Email – Home@PaulineLawson.co.uk

facebook.com/EmotionAllCoaching

twitter.com/emotionallserv

instagram.com/emotion_all_coaching

14

SHARON PORTER

HELPING PERINATAL WOMEN SELF IDENTIFY WHERE THEY ARE AT

What does Mental Health mean to you? Have you suffered from it? Do you know others suffering? Mental Health means different things to different people, take some time now to ask yourself what it means to you.

This epidemic has hit the UK hard creating a growing need for support. Mental health problems cost the UK economy an estimated £70–100 billion each year, with 1 in 4 adults experiencing a Mental Health problem. "The UK is not alone: The World Health Organisation predicts that by 2030 if we continue as we are, Mental Health problems will be the greatest health burden on humanity."

The more we can talk about the concerns anyone is having and lead with a proactive approach, the more we can help support them. In the last few years, I have seen a lot of local support groups grow from strength to strength showing the need for this type of peer support. Mixed anxiety and depression are the most common Mental Health disorder in Britain, with 7-8% of people meeting criteria for diagnosis.

My work centres around Pre and Postnatal Women, - So I am going to focus here on sharing facts and information on Perinatal Mental Health. The symptoms I will describe are very similar to Mental Health as a whole and are non-exhaustive.

Perinatal Mental Health covers the period during pregnancy and the first year after birth. Peri is the Latin term for 'around' and natal being the Latin term for 'birth'. Other terms used are Prenatal and Antenatal meaning before birth, during or relating to pregnancy, Postnatal, and Postpartum relates to the period after childbirth.

Examples of Perinatal Mental Health include:

Perinatal Depression (PD)

Perinatal Anxiety (PA)

Perinatal Obsessive Compulsive Disorder (POCD)

Perinatal Post Traumatic Stress Disorder (PPTSD)

Postnatal Psychosis (PP)

All the Perinatal Mental Illnesses fall into different ranges varying from mild, moderate to severe which in turn range in varying degree of treatment and care. "Around 1 in 5 women will experience a mental health problem during pregnancy or in the year after giving birth. This carries a total long-term cost to society of about £8.1 billion for each one-year of children born." It can happen to anyone, whether there is a history of mental illness or not. These stats show how huge the problem is and the impact it has on society.

I feel there is limited support towards mums-to-be and new mums regarding their emotional well-being during and after pregnancy. Pregnancy and the arrival of the new baby can be one of the happiest times in a woman's life but can also be a scary and stressful time, with a huge 30% of new mums never talking to a professional about their perinatal Mental Health problems. There are many changes physically and psychologically which place additional pressure on the new mum and the people around her, plus many other factors listed below.

- Concern about the details being noted on her medical records
- The stigma attached to Mental Health problems
- Not believing the health care professionals could or would help
- A risk it could prove the validity of her fears
- She thought it was normal
- She felt embarrassed or worried

- She thought her baby would be taken away
- A worry of being judged

Let's look at each of the Perinatal Mental Health examples in a little more detail.

Baby Blues (BB)

Baby Blues is a very common postnatal mental illness with as many as 60- 80% of new mums suffering with the condition. This is very short-lived compared to the other conditions, lasting for about 1 to 2 weeks after the arrival of your baby. No prescribed treatment is required for this, however talking about how you are feeling with friends or family may support you during this period of time.

Some typical symptoms may include:

*Extreme and rapid mood changes

*Frustration

*Exhaustion

*Unable to sleep or wanting to sleep all the time

*Irritable

*Feel trapped

*Overreacting

. . .

Perinatal Depression (PD)

Perinatal Depression is a much deeper and longer-term depression lasting for more than 2 weeks. It affects 15-20% of all new mums. Symptoms can present themselves suddenly or gradually at any time during the first few months to a year post-delivery.

Symptoms may include some of the following:

*Trouble feeling connected to your fetal baby

*Increased anxiety

*Low energy and fatigue

*Frequent crying or weepiness

*Sad & low mood

*Overwhelmed

*Worthless or guilty

*Increase or decrease in usual appetite

*Sleeping more or less than usual

*Extremely worried about your baby

*Uninterested in your newborn

*Uninterested in activities you once enjoyed

*Hopelessness

*Death and Suicidal thoughts

*Thoughts about harming someone or your baby

Hormonal changes are the most likely cause, although not yet proven of Postnatal Depression and Baby Blues. This is due to hormone levels of estrogen and progesterone dropping drastically within 48 hours of the baby's arrival after being very high during pregnancy. Couple these chemical changes with the physical and emotional changes of becoming a parent, along with any past Mental Health history issues and this increases your risk of suffering from PD and BB. Prolonged depression may be more harmful to mum and baby more so than the side effects of treatment and medications.

Perinatal Anxiety (PA)

Perinatal Anxiety is a heightened feeling of being unsafe or threatened and can present itself through your thoughts, emotional and physical feelings, and actions. Approximately 6% of pregnant women and 10% of all new mums experience anxiety.

Some of the following symptoms and actions may include:

*Worst-case scenario

*Unsettled sleep

*Increased heart rate

*Tight chest

*Reduced appetite

*Muscle tension

*Shallow breathing

*Reluctance to leave the house

*Avoiding seeing people

*Over controlling situations

*Heart palpitations

*Worry and panic

Perinatal Obsessive Compulsive Disorder (POCD)

Perinatal Obsessive Compulsive Disorder is a combination of OBSESSIONS - ANXIETY - COMPULSIONS, affecting 2 in 100 women in pregnancy and 2-3 in 100 women in the year after giving birth.

Symptoms may present as:

*Perfectionism

*Intense fear or worry

*A thought of harming someone

*Horrendous thoughts and visions that seem real

*Repetitive/rituals

*Depression

*Constant checking on the baby

Perinatal Post Traumatic Stress Disorder (PPTSD)

Perinatal Post Traumatic Stress Disorder may be experienced following shocking, unexpected and traumatic experiences during birth affecting 30 in 1,000 births.

Some of the characteristics can include:

*Flashbacks

*Nightmares

*Feeling detached

*Lack of concentration

*Panic attacks

*Self-destructive behaviour

*Irritability

*Keeping busy

*Postnatal depression

Postnatal Psychosis (PP)

Postnatal Psychosis is a mix of depression, mania, and psychosis, and is the most severe but rare condition, affecting 1-2 in 1,000 births. This can start as early as days or weeks after delivery.

Possible symptoms experienced:

*Hallucinations

*Delusions

*Suicidal thoughts

*Thoughts about harming your baby and/or yourself

*Paranoia or suspicious of other people

*Severe depression or manic

*Racing thoughts

*Being very confused

*Out of character behaviour

Katie's story (below) is an example of a first-hand perspective of Postnatal Psychosis. She was willing to share her experience to support other mums.

Game Changer

The birth of your first baby amazing right? When you hold them in your arms for the first time after 9 long-awaited months and look in their eyes for the first time you feel what can only be described as painstaking love for your beautiful little bundle of joy!

Wrong... for me anyway! Preconceived ideas of how this was supposed to be were blown out the water in seconds. In fact, the first time I looked in Hannah's eyes next to me in her little see-through cot I was not filled with love and happiness, I was petrified, alone and in a very dark place!

Her eyes were blue, but to me, they looked black and devilish. I didn't know this at the time, but this was the beginning of the hardest journey I would ever face.

Hannah was born via emergency C-section under a general anaesthetic, after an already traumatic labour and 9 months of hyperemesis gravidarum. Neither I nor my loving husband witnessed our daughter being born, which I think was the reason I suffered so much for the first 6 months of Hannah's life.

The most vivid memory I have of those days was when I was changing Hannah's nappy. She was laid on her changing mat. The baby laid there looked like a demon. I screamed for my husband, panicked, terrified and confused. I believed my little girl had been switched at the hospital, and the baby we had brought home with us was evil. I was scared to be alone with her, scared of the dark and terrified when her eyes met mine when I was breastfeeding. I planned (unbeknown to my husband) to leave one night, leaving Hannah with him and end my life because the alternative was far too terrifying. I now understand I was very ill, but those thoughts and visions will haunt me for the rest of my life.

I was diagnosed with postnatal psychosis when Hannah was a few weeks old. Rather than enjoying those first few early months like you're led to believe, the days were long, dark and filled with fear. I didn't believe Hannah was my little girl, she was something very evil in my eyes. The worst part being is that I didn't believe I was unwell. Luckily I had amazing support around me and the people who loved and cared about me the most knew something was very, very wrong. I started medication via my GP, which wasn't a quick fix but was definitely helping.

I heard about a class called "Buggy 4 Fitness" via a friend. To cut a long story very short, I reluctantly signed up. I packed up Hannah into the car screaming, and nervously took the first few steps to what I firmly believe saved me and my little girl.

We were met by Sharon who instantly put me and Hannah at ease. My fitness level was nonexistent, but Sharon assured me it didn't matter! All my anxieties about what I would do if Hannah cried, or I needed to breastfeed, or I simply fell into a heap on the floor all instantly melted away.

I was out in the fresh air with my baby, meeting other new mums, exercising and feeling like I could take on the world!

Buggy 4 Fitness was our saviour! I worked out come rain or shine, even in the snow and loved every second. Before I knew it, I was feeling better. I can never thank Sharon enough for offering an opportunity for mums to exercise with their baby's in a positive environment and share concerns and experiences. She will probably never realise how much she and these sessions helped me to bond with Hannah. Happy mum... happy baby!

I am still in touch with Sharon to this day and continued with her classes after I had my little boy Jack. Hannah who was then a toddler came with me and we all exercised together!

In summary, medication, of course, plays a part in the treatment of postnatal Mental Health, but exercising in the fresh air with your baby and a truly inspirational lady who pushes you just enough to reach your potential... well that's the game changer!

Thank you Sharon xx

This is why I am so passionate about marrying together fitness, Mental Health and wellbeing for not only women and men that are new to parenthood but everyone inclusively. I feel extremely touched after hearing how I impacted Katie's life and I want to continue making a positive difference within the lives of all that come in contact with me.

Men and Perinatal Mental Health

Perinatal Mental Health doesn't just affect women, 1 in 10 dads will become depressed during their partners pregnancy. Studies have found that half of men who have partners with postpartum depression will go on to develop it themselves. With 1 in 8 partners experiencing Mental Health problems and most receiving no support. Postnatal Depression in men can present itself from 3 to 6 months after birth. Men can have some of the symptoms mentioned in this chapter along with Mental Health as a whole, the symptoms are all very similar apart from a few differing symptoms which may include:

*Marital conflict

*Fear & confusion

*Indecisiveness

*Negative parenting behaviours

It's important to ask for help if you notice anything mentioned, it's not a sign of weakness or something to feel guilty about.

Think back to my opening paragraph - What does Mental Health mean to you? Have you suffered with it?

Now ask yourself, how have you been feeling lately?

Following the NICE guidelines ask yourself the questions below:

During the past month, have you often been bothered by feeling down, depressed or hopeless?

During the past month, have you often been bothered by having little interest or pleasure in doing things?

Over the last two weeks, how often have you been bothered by feeling nervous, anxious or on edge?

Over the last two weeks, how often have you been bothered by not being able to stop or control worrying?

If you answered positively to any of the above questions, reach out to your GP, midwife or health visitor. After you have sought the appropriate help, we look below at ways to maintain Positive Mental Health, this being inclusive to wellbeing as a whole. You may find some ideas here that you can fit into your daily routine.

Positive Mental Health

Looking after your Mental Health is about being proactive in your approach for your whole wellbeing, starting as early as preconception leading through your postnatal years. There are several facets to wellbeing, and this is broken down into 5 specific sections. They all interlink and connect.

Mental Wellbeing ** Physical Wellbeing ** Spiritual Wellbeing **

Emotional Wellbeing ** Social Wellbeing

Mental Wellbeing - The condition and healthiness of the mind

- Journal - writing a daily diary
- Talk more - friends, family, strangers

- Music - create and listen to your own feel good playlist
- Negative Self Talk - What self-defeating talk do you use? Make a list and then think of a positive alternative or coping thought
- Negative thoughts to positive thoughts
- Laugh
- Focus and purpose - Is there anything new you want to learn, arrange your own meet up, read, draw.

Physical Wellbeing - The condition and healthiness of the body

- Exercise - Sports (netball, hockey, dance, tennis), join a gym, join an organised class, cycle
- Be more active - Walking, take the stairs rather than the lift, jump off the bus a stop earlier, stretching, take a swim.
- Get out in nature - walk barefoot, explore the woods, gardening
- Nutrition - Eat a balanced diet, reduce caffeine and alcohol intake.
- Set goals - daily, weekly, monthly, long term
- Sleep - Aim for 6-8hours or take cat naps through the day
- Hydration - On average drink 2 litres of water a day.

Spiritual Wellbeing - defined as a sense of peace and contentment stemming from an individual's relationship with the spiritual aspects of life

- Mindfulness - Be present, the here and now. Apps - Breathe, Headspace, Insight Timer.
- Affirmations are positive statements that can help you to overcome self-sabotaging and negative thoughts. Feel the glow, have created some wonderful pregnancy affirmation cards.
- Meditation found on cd's, apps and YouTube.
- Positive Imagery and visualisation

Emotional Wellbeing associated with thoughts, feelings and behavioural responses.

- Knowing your own body and your feelings - Each month we go through cycles:-

- Menstruation
- Moon

- What's normal for you?
- How do you feel right now? Choose 3 descriptive words and write them down.
- Be kind to yourself
- Remember your good points

- Recognise your triggers

Social Wellbeing - Your sense of belonging and connection to family, friends, community, and groups.

- Plan activities/groups to attend through pregnancy and after the baby has arrived
- Create and respect your own boundaries
- Make it clear to people how they can help
- Find a support network of women at the same stage as you - Conceiving - Pregnancy - Postnatal
- Build connections and relationships
- Stay connected

If you could make one change to your life from each of the above areas, what would they be? Do you feel you could make improvements in any particular area? What would be the advantages to making a change? What would be the disadvantages?

Possible Solutions

My solution to the problem would be to have more thorough care throughout pregnancy and the postnatal period. Professions need to ask the correct questions and give education and information right from the moment they realise they are pregnant. Detailing tools and guidelines to help women self-identify their feelings and not allow anyone to think it's all part and parcel of becoming a new parent.

There are lots of hormonal changes but knowing what to look out for, what's normal and what's not, would keep them one step ahead. Attendance at fitness classes, include a pre health questionnaire which should be filled out prior to participation, likewise questionnaires as such could be implemented routinely at antenatal and post-natal appointments, Questionnaires such as the NHS Mood Self-Assessment Quiz (MSAQ), Edinburgh Post-natal Depression Scale (EPDS) and The Mood Disorder Questionnaire (MDQ) are examples of screening tools that are currently used.

Although these tools are available, a staggering 40% of the UK's services have no specialist perinatal Mental Health provision which shows the prevalence of the problem. However, NHS England has committed since 2016 to improving access to specialist perinatal Mental Health support by 30,000 women in all areas of England by 2020/21.

Create your circle of support - List who you would reach out to for each of the wellbeing sections. Who could you turn to for help with the housework? For help with child-care? For laughter?

If you have a positive Mental Health, based on the infor-mation, how can you help others? If we can all increase our awareness and recognise some of the signs we can guide each other to the care and support needed at the earliest time. The hardest step is the first.

When self-help may not be enough, ask for help! There is no one size fits all approach, it's what works for YOU the individual. That's why it's so important to take your own wellbeing into your own hands and find your tribe, in my fit family I help women feel strong, confident and happy in themselves throughout pregnancy, after the arrival of children and beyond.

SHARON PORTER

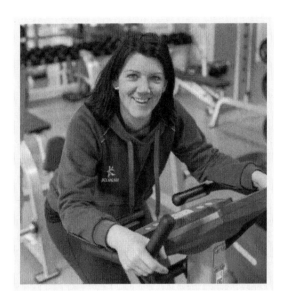

Sharon Porter is a fun filled, well-travelled, health and fitness go getter.

She is the founder of Buggy 4 Fitness and Sharon Porter Fitness.

Sharon has always loved exercise and sport - having taken part in just about any physical activity available to her since childhood.

As well as being on the football, netball, hockey and rugby teams at school, she fell in love with Karate and represented her country in the sport. Her black belt martial arts skills form some of her training programmes today.

It wasn't difficult for her to decide what career path to take - she has spent more than two decades gaining qualifications and working in the fitness industry in and around West Yorkshire.

Her expertise includes working with pregnant women, new mums and children. She also specialises in postnatal assessment and core restore. Diet and nutrition play a part in her teachings which clearly forms part of healthy living.

Her Qualifications range from L3 Award in Designing Pre and Post Natal Exercise Programmes, L2 ITEC & YMCA Fitness Instruction, L2 Instructing Health Related Exercise for Children, L3 Advanced Fitness Instruction, L3 Nutrition and Weight Management, Adv CPD in Postnatal Assessment, Core Restore and Functional Exercise Programming.

Her mission is to enrich and help change people's lives for the better. To help women reconnect with themselves in mind, body and spirit during and after the arrival of children.

She wants to be able to contribute and give back in a big way and wants to see what she is truly capable of.

Contact:

Website: www.sharonporter.org.uk

Email: hello@sharonporter.org.uk

15

VIVIENNE RAWNSLEY

"*N*o, I don't love you and haven't for some time".

My heart thudded in my chest like it never had before as I stared at my husband's emotionless face. Was I hearing right? No. I mustn't have woken up properly yet. Whilst I'd known things hadn't been perfect, what relationship is? I hadn't had any clue that his love for me had gone. And just like that, he was gone. He left behind 17 years of marriage just like that.

I spent the whole day ironing, a task that I hate. Over the duration of that weekend, I lost over half a stone in weight. What was I going to do? Divorce was something that happened to other people, not me! I had five little boys that needed a mum and dad together in a loving home. My entire world had fallen apart in one day.

All I could think about was how I was going to fix it?

Until that moment I had always believed I could fix anything; from saving the runt of the rabbit litter by feeding it with milk from my finger all night, to rescuing my sister from bullies by having a fight with a girl and ending up with my black coat being strewn with copious amounts of my detached blonde tresses.

I had to be able to fix this too.

I lost even more weight, had my hair cut into a new trendy style, wore the most alluring clothing and even went out to buy the latest in wedge heeled shoes to make my legs look longer but with no avail. He had met someone new, and no amount of effort on my part would get him to come home and try again. My self-esteem was at an all-time low. For the first time, I felt I didn't know who I was or where I was heading and I was overwhelmed with a sense of failure.

From this episode in my life, I went on a mission to prove to myself, and the world that I was good enough. I registered on a couple of dating sites, driving up and down the length of Britain to meet around 80 random strangers in motorway services, pubs, and restaurants to fulfil my quest. I was trying to boost my self-esteem but this ultimately left me feeling empty and further rejected.

Attending dance classes 4 or 5 times a week and joining a scuba diving training club were other hobbies I engaged in to prove that I was acceptable and that I was enough. Constantly hoping that the affirmation from others would fill that void inside. Although I became an accomplished dancer and qualified in scuba diving it, was still not enough.

I set up a business that after a very successful launch failed. I know now this was because I undervalued myself and gave a low entry price to those who were struggling financially. More failure for me to swallow. Another drop in my self-esteem. I had to carry on moving forward though as I had my five sons to keep going for.

In an attempt to maintain the lifestyle they had grown accustomed to, I took my sons on ski holidays that were way outside my tax credit budget and so the search to being complete and whole again continued.

Life had challenges, but I never gave up trying to make it better. I was always looking for a solution, a way to feel better, to feel truly happy and at peace. Then one day, whilst in the shopping area at Manchester airport, I came across two books that sparked my interest, Fiona Harold's 'Be Your Own Life Coach' and Ken Robinson's 'Finding your Element: How to Discover Your Talents and Passions and Change your Life.' Lying on a sunbed in Tenerife, I read these books and was inspired to embark upon the next chapter of my life.

I enrolled in a Personal Performance Coaching training and an NLP course. I believed I was on my way, the courses were going to fix me, and make me whole and complete again.

I excelled in the courses and passed with flying colours yet I didn't feel any better about myself. On the inside, the feeling of unworthiness remained. So my journey into personal development continued for several years, me spending days on end and weekends away from home, thousands of pounds and hundreds of hours doing course after course trying to find that part of me that was missing. Searching for the person who could fix and fill that need inside me.

Years later, with a plethora of knowledge and certificates to prove I was good enough, I realised that no external source was going to fill the void I had deep within me. It was like a light bulb suddenly lit up inside my head and I realised I needed to stop searching and actually just be still and connect with myself. I discovered that everything I needed was inside me, that I was enough already.

But where had the story of me come from? I pondered upon what had happened to me in my life to leave me thinking that I wasn't enough? Where had the need to prove that I was enough originated? Was it actually from my divorce or was it from other earlier experiences or incidences in my life?

As I reflected, I remembered incidences at home as the big sister when I felt that I hadn't achieved what was expected of me. I remembered times at school when I had felt that I didn't fit in and even when I tried hard to fit in by wearing the same clothes as others did and hanging out with the less 'swotty' group that need to be enough was lacking.

I remembered early feelings of rejection when the boys I fancied never liked me, the ones who did, I felt obligated to be interested in them. I always felt as though I had to seem to be being perfect in order to be enough. The real me just got squashed deeper and deeper inside, squeezing out in rebellious moments and ending up doing seemingly crazy things.

How had this happened? I was from a 'normal' family with loving parents who worked hard to provide everything they could for me and my sister and brother. We lived in a comfortable home, ate good food – my mum is an awesome cook even though my dad's turkey carcass soup was always questionable- and even had hotel holidays abroad in the days when many people never even left the country, let alone stay in hotels.

I passed the 11+ selection exam and went on to achieve O' levels, A' levels, and a degree so had the credentials to be accepted as intelligent. I had been highly regarded by the Principle and lecturers at college and senior leadership teams in my career in education.

I had given birth to five healthy sons and always maintained a fit and healthy body reducing my weight to my starting point after each pregnancy. Looking in on my life from the outside, I appeared to be a successful high achiever, yet on the inside, I felt totally unfulfilled.

I had got lost in the story that I had created around past events, and the interpretation that I had made of them, that left me in a place of lack, feeling unworthy and not being enough. It was realising this that made a huge difference to how I feel inside. The past isn't real. It's gone and how we choose to recall it is up to us.

When I was little I remember my dad telling me bedtime stories at night. My favourites were the ones that he made up about three mischievous puppies called 'Woof', 'Tuff' and 'Snuff' and the adventures that they got up to. Each night's stories would be different unless I asked for an adventure being repeated and even then there were adaptations depending on what my dad remembered and what he felt like putting into the story that night. Sometimes if it was raining outside the story would take place on a rainy day and if it was a birthday so the story would be based around a birthday.

Remembering these stories got me thinking. What if the experiences in my life I'd remembered, like the stories from long before, were having an impact on how I'd remembered the event or incident? With the way I was feeling or the things that had been happening at the time and then like a story I'd made it up?

I'd made up who I was based on what I thought I had to be and what I thought others thought of me. I then realised if I had made it up, I was the author of the story and could rewrite it in a different way. In fact, I could create my life and the story of my life in any way I chose to.

That point in time began my journey into finding me. I'd had sessions with several counsellors. I engaged in EMDR (Eye Movement Desensitisation Reprogramming), and put a new perspective on elements of my past and removed blame from those who maybe I'd felt had let me down or impacted on me in a negative way in the past.

CBT (Cognitive Behavioural Therapy) group sessions were provided by the local health authority during which I felt that all I was doing was engaging in the challenges that others were dealing with. I even had hypnotherapy and not knowing what to expect or being informed about it prior to the sessions didn't feel I'd experienced it and was left feeling conned.

Now I'm not saying that these are not really useful and well-proven systems that work. For some people, they are very effective and life-changing. It's important to remember at this point, I am the eldest daughter of three children, I am creative, I am resilient and I like to maintain control over what's going on around me because that gives me a feeling of safety and being ok, and will use this to hide out physically or metaphorically when my inner self feels scared or threatened.

So what was I going to do? How was I going to get out of this vicious circle, the repeating pattern of victimhood and the life that really wasn't working for me in the way that I wanted it to?

I needed to start telling myself a different story! I also realised I needed to stop running away from my feelings and face them head-on.

Did you know that the heart, the part of us that feels pain, is stronger than the brain, the most powerful source of electro-magnetic energy in the human body, producing the largest rhythmic electromagnetic field of any of the body's organs? In fact, the heart's electrical field is about 100 times greater in amplitude than the electrical activity generated by the brain and 5000 times stronger magnetically? So if that is true, which scientists say it is, why was I concentrating so much on what was going on in my continuing negative thought patterns? Why was I not focussing more on my feelings?

Those parts of me that had been dumbed and numbed down so much, that when an assessor from the Mental Health service asked me how I felt about what was going on, I was unable to answer her. Or more accurately, I wouldn't allow myself that vulnerability because it might hurt too much and rip open the scars that were still tender.

Instead, I talked about my external situation and what other people in my life were doing. If I was to put the past in the past and rewrite my story, then I needed to start doing things in a different way, start acknowledging those feelings that my huge electronic magnetic power-house was pulsating into every cell in my body.

So how did I start? What did I do?

Nelson Mandela said that, "There is no easy walk to freedom anywhere, and many of us will have to pass through the valley of the shadow of death again and again before we reach the mountaintop of our desires".

My first step up my mountain was that I acknowledged where I was at. Instead of looking externally to find the easy route, the usual brave face I put on for myself and anyone else looking in, it was time to explore how I really was, what I felt and the feelings that I wanted to experience rather than those I had created stories around that were expected or allowed.

I had a table filled with certificates that proved my skill set, I had my five boys who grew from those not so tiny babies into men bigger and stronger than me. I had a house overfilled with possessions. A regular income that was always overstretched.

I had attended hundreds of hours and spent thousands of pounds attending personal development, business and speaker training. All of them shouting in loud voices my need for external evidence to prove who I was ,and yet never really representing the me that is beneath the surface.

I began to realise that unless I looked beneath the superficial and continued to rely on the ability of others to fix me, I would never allow the past to diminish and the essence of me to rise like a phoenix from the ashes.

The next step was creating space. Space to feel. A space that removed the noise of the could do, should do, have to. A space that would allow the desire that was shelved somewhere inside me to grow.

I started to take time for me. As a full-time teacher, homemaker and carer of 5 boys, the balls I juggled were many and the time I took for me {slim}.

However, I began to take a bath in the morning instead of a shower. To make myself and drink, cups of a wide variety of delicious herbal teas. To download audible books to listen to whilst I was driving in the car. I created opportunities to explore where I was at, what I was actually enjoying. What I was feeling satisfied with and what was adding to the pressures and burdens of the day.

And as I felt, something amazing happened. I began to explore the reality of my life, the facts about what really existed, versus the stories that I had created way back when. I didn't even have origins for many of them, just vague recollections of how it might have been and from the interpretations I'd made in my formative years. This explained how my perceived identity had been born.

The eldest daughter. I knew what it was like for me when I had my first son, that unknown realm of parenthood. How did I do it? Would someone come and take him from me now I'd done the carrying him for 9+ months and given birth to him? Surely, I wasn't going to be trusted with this tiny human being? What had it been like for my parents?

How had it been being the eldest of three children?

When had things been said in fun and not, that I'd taken to heart and made my reality?

What events had taken place that I had made my own interpretation about? Where I'd created who I was, what I was worth and capable of?

Why would my creative imagination have been any less vivid then?

I remembered being at school and being asked to write a story, being given the title and then being allowed to write whatever I wanted. If I could write whatever I wanted then what was so different about now? Was it possible that when I woke up in the morning, rather than the day taking charge of the way I felt and the things I accomplished, I could design the day and the way I felt?

Better still, could I create a plan from the things I wanted to accomplish, to support the way I wanted to feel and fit them around the things that were expected of me? And could I even explore those things that were expected of me? Were they really expected of me or had I made those boundaries too? And if I had made them, then I could then also, unmake or alter them? Just like the eraser in my pencil case when I was at school, I could rub out the parts of my life and the parts of me that were leaving me with negative feelings and rewrite my story and create a new plan for my life moving forward.

It was at this point that I revisited hypnotherapy, however this time as a practitioner rather than as a client. I learned about the power of the subconscious mind, and that how although logically and cognitively I could know about all the memories, thoughts and feelings I wanted to rub out, alter and change, part of me kept holding on tightly not letting go and allowing me to transform my life.

My subconscious mind. The part of me that has always been awake, always been working hard to keep me alive and keep me safe. Storing the memories and events of the past as a reminder of what is dangerous and what is safe and how I must behave accordingly.

Through my period of training, I was always the person to volunteer for any new technique or process to be demonstrated and practiced with 'clients' between training sessions. As I continued being the subject of hypnosis and using hypnosis with others I started to notice changes taking place.

My subconscious letting go of the patterns of the past and rebooting with programmes that allow me freedom and choice. Ways that I would have reacted to situations previously being different, things that would have upset, disturbed or angered me in the past having little or no effect. My feelings around situations of the past were diminished. Transformation was taking place.

This continued over time, creating the space I desired to start doing things differently, having the opportunity to choose how I react and instead respond to situations. The old thought patterns of the past no-longer taking charge. Allowing me the space to acknowledge my feelings about situations and make choices rather than living on auto-pilot.

Clients too began to notice deep and profound changes taking place in their lives. Those who had suffered from the feelings of depression for most of their lives, recognising that the feelings had lifted. Leaving them with good and not so good days but no longer feeling depressed.

Other clients overcame feelings of anxiety that had been created in their formative years. Leaving them enjoying newfound confidence and ability to communicate effectively with others, create relationships and make career choices that would have previously seemed impossible.

The impact of the use of hypnosis blended with the other skills I have developed over the years was creating tangible differences in my life and the lives of those I worked with.

One client worked through the limiting physical conditions of fibromyalgia, underactive thyroid and diabetes. She also overcame the emotional limiting beliefs of not being worthy and not being good enough resulting in her being able to lose over four stone in weight. This meant she achieved her goal of having knee replacements so she could go for long walks in the countryside once more. Another client conquered their stories, fears and limiting beliefs to being appointed in the job of their dreams. Many clients de-cluttered and discarded emotional as well as physical baggage that they no-longer-needed or felt was necessary for them to hold onto.

So my life began to change. I began to make new choices. No longer feeling the need to please others because I was the big sister, the wife, the ex-wife, the mother ... but being free to choose, free to write my story in whichever and whatever way I chose. Creating a successful business that supports others in recognising the stories that they tell themselves, changing stories and transforming lives.

It's interesting that I find myself sitting writing this chapter in the same place that my journey began, in Tenerife. Another of those opportunities that would never have happened without the changes that have taken place in me.

In the words of Rumi, 'What you seek, is seeking you.'

Once upon a time, there lived a girl called Cinderella...

And the beautiful princess lived happily ever after.

The End

AUTHOR BIO

VIVIENNE RAWNSLEY

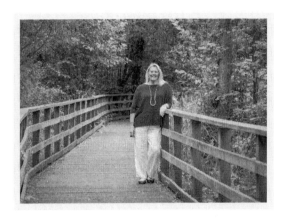

Becoming a single mum to five sons was the beginning of a journey into personal development, more specifically the development of Vivienne.

A lover of learning, that during her years at school hit peaks and troughs, has enabled Vivienne to gain a number of qualifications and accreditations, most notably as a Clinical Hypnotherapist and Psychotherapist, a Neuro-Linguistic Programming Practitioner and Precision Personal Performance Coach.

Utilising these and other skills inside a blended

approach, Vivienne brings focussed transformation programmes to her face-to-face and online group workshops, bespoke packages to her one-to-one clients and exclusive and luxury retreats to those who prefer to get away from it all and indulge themselves in immersive, reset opportunities.

As an international transformation coach and hypnotherapist, Vivienne has a passion for making a difference in the lives of others, taking them from overwhelm, stress, fear, disconnection and anxiety to happiness, freedom, joy, fulfilment, and ease.

Previous clients have said:

'I was very skeptical at first but after a few sessions I feel more confident, relaxed and empowered.'

'Vivienne has helped me become the person I've always wanted to be.'

'Through hypnosis, Vivienne has helped me so much with my confidence and self-acceptance. She has enabled me to live my life more freely.'

Recently Vivienne has featured as a panellist at Shaa Wasmund MBE National Women's Conference, Co-Authored a Bestselling Book and presented training at the Great Yorkshire Showground Wonderful World of Wellbeing Event together with other local and national personal development, education and business events.

With a background of over thirty years in mainstream and special education, both as a member of senior leadership teams, classroom practitioner and leadership trainer and facilitator, Vivienne blends her knowledge of working in highly pressured result-driven environments together with her in-depth knowledge of the creation of identity, and the freedom we can experience when we explore what is possible outside the limitations that the past has imposed on us.

In her free time Vivienne enjoys travelling at home and abroad, clocking thousands of miles onto her odometer, dancing under the stars, swimming in the sea, upcycling tattered treasures in creative ways, indulging in delicious food, spending time with her family, and is happiest when she is based close to the sea on hot sunny days.

To connect with Vivienne, you can find her at

www.viviennerawnsley.com

viv@viviennerawnsley.com

 facebook.com/viviennerawnsley

 instagram.com/viviennerawnsley

16

WAYNE EVANS

THE POWER OF FOCUS

$\mathcal{M}$y childhood was good, we had everything we needed in life; clothes, toys and a nice house. We were just a normal, working class family.

My auntie and uncle lived two doors down which is where I spent most of my younger days growing up with my older cousin. On the weekend I would always be with him going fishing. We would always have such a good time and laugh all the way home in his old ford fiesta!

I believe my starting point to a downward journey started when my uncle had a heart attack and died at the age of fifty. I remember the whole event very clearly as my auntie ran up the street screaming "Help me, Help me" at the top of her voice. There was absolute panic in the house with my auntie screaming and crying loudly.

My mom put me, my brother and sister in her bed out the way so we didn't see anything.

I was twelve years old at the time, so old enough to understand what was going on but not old enough to process the events properly. I took care of my younger brother and sister and got them to sleep whilst all the chaos was going on downstairs. Once everything settled down my mom came upstairs and explained that my uncle had died from a heart attack. I remember bursting out in tears. My world felt as though it had turned upside down, this was the first time I encountered death.

Growing up I shared my weekends with my nan and my cousin. If I wasn't fishing, I was down my nan and grandads playing in the garden trying to catch birds with homemade traps or playing in the tool shed! I used to get up early with my nan and go to the local markets most of the day before coming home to watch Saturday evening TV. Sunday was the best day as my nan always cooked the best Sunday dinner! My nan and I were close. She used to hug and kiss me all the time and she would always go out her way for me or anyone really. She was a kind warm hearted person who helped anyone even if she didn't know them.

As I grew into a teenager, I stopped going down my nan's and started going out with my school friends. It just wasn't cool to go down your grandparents when I could hang around with my friends and play football etc. I recall the night the house phone rang and watching my mom answer it and turn white. She was told to get down my nan's house as she had just had a heart attack. It was clear to see from returning home my nan had died, and it was devastating news.

That moment changed my life. A deep sense of guilt ran over me!

I stopped going down to see my nan on the weekends to play with out with my friends. It was probably the last time I cried without having any control to stop. Inside I was absolutely furious with myself because I stopped going down to see her. The funeral was one of the hardest things I have ever had to do. To watch my mom break down in tears absolutely killed me and added to the guilt. There is one thing in life you should not see and that is your mom breaking down.

At the funeral, I believed I had to put a brave face on that day to stay strong for my mom. I was thirteen years old and bottled all the emotions up that day without shedding a tear. Later that day in the car driving back home my dad turned to my mom and said, "Don't worry you'll get over it!". My mom was so emotionally drained that day she never gave a thought about what my dad had just said to her as she had just buried her mom. This was clear sign of what had been going on behind closed doors!

Things went from bad to worse as my dad slept in the

spare room and they were fighting regularly. I recall walking in from school and my mom was broken hearted at the kitchen table. She sat me down and explained that my dad had left us to be with another woman! Again, my world had just been turned upside down only six months after losing my nan whilst riddled with guilt I now felt unwanted by my dad. It was then I recalled a memory from a few months earlier – Driving round with my mom late at night spying on my dad!

Life became tough without my dad as we had no income coming in. We went from having full cupboards of food to the bare minimum buying all the cheap crap from Netto! I was a very tall lad and every start of term I was told, "Do not ruin these school trousers they need to last all year!". The only problem was that after a few months they were up my ankles like Michael Jackson trousers! Not very cool at all!

My dad signed the house over to my mom which I thought was good of him. It was 5 years later we found out he had forged my mom's signature all the insurances were signed over to him and worth a lot more than the house. When my dad was asked would you like weekend access towards your kids my dad replied, "No, but can I have the dog!". Those were the exact words he used in court! How do you cope at thirteen years old losing your uncle, your nan you grew up with, your parents splitting up and your dad choosing a dog over his kids – all in less than twenty four months?

My schooling was going downhill fast because of my home life. My interest in school was non existence and I found myself rebelling. I was angry inside which lead to constant fighting at school, being expelled regularly and being in the wrong crowd. The anger was topped off listening to my mom crying downstairs before she came to bed each night. I was completely out of control, getting told many times that I would amount to nothing.

To make things completely worse I met some friends that smoked weed. We used to smoke it during our dinner break on the school field. My friends went around this local house where they got the weed from and introduced me to the dealer. We got on really well and over the next few months I spent a lot of time around the house having a smoke and a drink.

I met some really interesting people to say the least as the house was like an open house where people used to drop in at anytime of the day or night! I remember being introduced to a guy who always had something up his sleeve! He kept putting his hand to his mouth. I used to look at him thinking, "What the hell is he doing?". When he trusted me after a few weeks he explained he sniffed gas and asked, "Do you want to try it?". I thought this looks pretty cool why not! So we went to the shop and I brought my first can of gas!

I took the cap off and sucked the gas up! It was a very weird sensation at first but after a few weeks I could see why he did it. As I got more trusted with the dealer, spending more time around the house I was asked if I would like to bag up some amphetamine (Speed). I thought I was some sort of gangster opening up the drug bags and spooning the drugs into the smaller bags and weighing them out! As the weeks rolled by I was left alone to do the bagging up and was always rewarded with a bag for the weekend.

I met up with a friend and explained I could get speed anytime. He brought up in conversation that he also has been taking speed but had a much better way of taking it. I was intrigued! "How many ways are there?" I asked. He explained that he had been injecting it and the rush was something else, much better than putting it on your tongue. I had mixed feelings of excitement! I knew it wrong, but the temptation was so bad that I had to just try it at least once!

We met at our local primary school in a very secluded spot. When he pulled the needle out I shit myself! I thought, "Wayne what the hell are you doing?". On the other hand, I really wanted to experience the buzz. My friend put a belt around my arm and found a vein! I was so nervous; it was a very surreal moment! He pieced my skin and pushed the needle in, slowly pressing the top of the syringe downwards.

Wow! My friend was right! The buzz was out of this world! After a few hours of chatting rubbish to each other we parted ways and walked home. This meeting happened twice more over the next few weeks and I enjoyed it! I only stopped after I had a big telling off from a friend of mine called Marie Purcell, who I'd confided in at school about injecting and sniffing gas.

I did my exams and walked away with absolutely no grades whatsoever. My mom to this day does not know what fully went on with my disastrous end to school. Once I finished school I spent all my time down the dealer's house. We were at raves all over the UK regularly taking high amounts of ecstasy tablets, LSD, amphetamines and high strength lager every weekend. I feel like I had been groomed into having a relationship with the dealer because at the time I had only just turned sixteen and she was twenty six.

If a man twenty six was giving free drugs to a girl who had just turned sixteen whilst sleeping together there would be a massive uproar in 2019! Over the next twelve months I did some really stupid things that I deeply regret. Drink and drug driving, locked up in a police cell for fighting on the streets and we even planned a burglary at a post office with the local thief - but thankfully it never came off! We had some really fun times and I met some very interesting people, but everything revolved around drink and drugs, but once that was taken away there was no common ground between us.

Things started turning bad and abusive. She had a very

vicious temper made worse with jealous emotions mixed with drink. I recall a time before Christmas we were having a few drinks at a local pub. I got chatting to an old school friend who worked behind the bar. I sat down and went to take a sip of my beer when pint glasses flew past my face! Followed by another and another! "I've seen you talking to her", she yelled. I stood up and walked out biting my tongue thinking, "Wayne just walk away before you do something stupid". I walked to her house trying my hardest to calm down when suddenly she pulled up in a taxi. She got out the taxi and started yelling at me whilst punching me in the face.

In a split second I lashed out and hit the window on her front door putting my hand completely through it! What a big mistake, the window had wire in the glass! I sliced my hand completely open and bled everywhere. We went inside to try and stop the bleeding but it wasn't working so she called the ambulance. There was a chunk of flesh an inch long on the floor that had dropped off! I went to the hospital that night and received sixteen stitches in my right hand but more importantly, I knew it was over and time to change. She was a good person deep down with good heart who would give strangers her last bit of change if they needed it. We had some fantastic times but it was time for me to grow up and stop this lifestyle.

I found a job working in a factory but still lived a poor lifestyle going to the pub each night. I was drinking alcohol and smoking cannabis on my lunch break, I desperately needed help. I noticed a kickboxing gym on my way home and decided out of the blue to get off the bus and take a look. I was greeted by a very intimidating looking Jamaican guy with a gold tooth called "Blacka". I decided to give it a go and promised to be there next week.

To my surprise I was the only white guy in the gym, and I thought, "What the hell am I doing here!". After doing some basics I heard, "get your sparring kit on!" My first ever session and I am sparring; what the hell! I got knocked from pillar to post with some students doing jumping kicks on me. I walked outside to find my head spinning and feeling sick! However, in a completely weird way I thought to myself, "I bloody loved that!".

I continued to go for another three months really enjoying it. My training got cut short due to starting a new job so I found another gym. This was when I met the most influential man and the person who I owe a great deal of gratitude towards, Mr Dave Hlyton. I started training and loved it! I finally found a male role model to look up to and model myself on. He was a true professional who only lived for training and his family. This guy changed my life!

I recall my first experience of Dave's ways being told, "There is a tournament down London next Sunday and you are fighting". I said, "Yeah let's go for it!". Inside I could have cried because I had only been training three months and I did not have a clue what I was doing. However Dave knew exactly what he was doing, testing me!

That tournament down in Windsor is where I experienced what the magic was all about. In my individual category I lost easily to someone who had more experience. I was just glad it was over in all honesty. The day was nearly over when Dave said, "Why don't you do the team event?". I thought, "Go on then at least I am lined up with some of my teammates" We came third and I received my first ever trophy... I was hooked!

I remember taking my little trophy to the gym to show the rest of the class, proud as punch, only to be struck by a young kid called Tony Davis. He was stood there with three belts around his waist having his photo took by the local newspaper. At the age of 15 yrs. old he was knocking grown men out! I just stared at him and thought, "Wow I want a belt around my waist". That moment I had discovered my motivation and purpose. I decided in my head I was going to win a kickboxing belt for my nan as a way of saying sorry for stopping going to see her before she died.

We spent six years up and down the country every Sunday competing in national tournaments. My life had flipped upside down from raves, taking class A drugs - to fighting in tournaments. My dream was to have a belt around my waist and make my nan proud of me.

We travelled across Europe to compete in countries such as Ireland, France and Belgium. I even represented my country at the world championships in Switzerland and Italy! Finally, after six years of constant travelling and fighting I got noticed and we got the call to fight for a Vacant European Kickboxing title in Dublin, Ireland. I trained like a man possessed! Every training session I put my heart and soul into it, total focus of lifting that belt for my nan. My dream was close!

We travelled over to Dublin all kitted out in our club tracksuits, for the first time ever we all looked the same, representing our club and country on the European stage. The feeling was absolutely amazing, as we were such a tiny club doing big things. We arrived at the venue to see all the belts laid out on the table, I said to myself, "That is my belt", over and over in my head as I walked around admiring the massive venue.

My walk out music came on. I walked to the ring fully focused and ready to give my heart and soul, losing was not an option. I climbed through the ropes and just stared at my opponent, ready for war. The bell rang and I hit him as hard as I could to see what his reaction would be. He backed off!

I knew from that punch I was too strong for him. I bullied him, round after round he did not want to know!

The final bell rang and we embraced each other with respect. We both knew I'd won the fight, but in his home town anything could happen! It was the longest, most agonising wait I had ever felt.

The ref held both our hands and I just closed my eyes and looked down. The wait was over. My hand went up! I'd done it! My dream of becoming European Champion had come true! The guilt over my nan which I had held on to for all those years had gone in an instant.

We were in the local papers when we got back home and I felt like a local celebrity. I loved it, I was doing something positive. A few months passed and we were back in full swing training again with our eyes focused on the World Cup in Italy, a massive prize. This was without doubt the toughest competition in Europe, if not the world.

There were only four fighters and one parent for this trip. We arrived at the airport proudly wearing our small club tracksuit representing club and country. We must have been the only fighters at the tournament without a sponsor! We loved the feeling of the being the underdogs as it boosted us up. We landed in Milan and the temperature was 35 degrees, with a daunting 200 mile trip to the hotel. I knew this was going to be a tough weekend but that temperature just made it a hell of a lot tougher!

Saturday morning we thought we were really clever travelling to the weigh in early. Sadly, so did a few thousand other fighters thinking the same thing! It was hot, sweaty and crowded as fighters got undressed to get weighed in.

Finally we got weighed in and found our allocated area in the main room that absolutely reeked of sweat and tiger balm. There were no proper toilets in our part of the venue, only holes in the floor that you had to squat down to use! It was no fun waiting in 35 degrees heat, with hundreds of people in the queue before you all going to the same holes in the ground. Welcome to the toughest tournament in Europe!

We got settled and set up our area where we could stretch, warm up and channel our focus ready to compete. There were over a hundred fighters in my category and my name was called out pretty much at the start. The nerves kicked in as I walked on the mat.

Mass amounts of sweat dripped down my back from nerves and the heat. I started brightly and took the lead, definitely growing in confidence throughout the fight. As the fight went on my nerves settled and I won the fight. The next five fights throughout the day went the same way as I grew more and more in confidence.

However, I did notice this Croatian guy just taking everyone out with his long arms and legs. He must have been six foot six tall, towering over everyone even me - and I am six foot two! The guy used being tall to his advantage, and he used it well, what made matters even worse was he was pretty aggressive too!

It was 5:30pm and I had made the semi-final against a shorter, but stocky powerful Italian fighter who had some fantastic kicks. I had been fighting on and off the mat for seven hours in 35 degree heat! Mentally and physically it had been the most challenging experience I have ever had to do. In the back of my mind though I knew if I could just get past this guy, I would be in the final of a world championship!

I started very nervously losing four points in a row having a panic! My nerves were getting the better of me and I lost the first round. My instructor gave me a roasting! It was just what I needed to hear! I started the second round on my toes, fired up and ready to go to war. I battled back to level the score and suddenly out of nowhere I landed a head kick taking me two points ahead!

There were thirty seconds on the clock and I just ran from him using all the dirty tricks in the book by simply stepping off the mat to waste time. It was not in my nature of fighting to hit and run, but I didn't care because the boy from Dudley was in a World championship final in Italy!

After ten hours it all boiled down to me and the big Croatian guy in the final. This time I started much better going into the second round two points up. The sweat just poured out of me with the heat and nerves, the conditions were tough. I ducked and got caught with a head kick.

The fight was tied with thirty seconds to go! Seven years of hard training came down to thirty seconds of fighting. I caught him with a jab and went one point ahead. His coach shouted at him and he just charged at me! I hit him with a right hand and the ref scored it to go two clear with ten seconds to go. I ran for dear life, wasting valuable seconds watching every second on the clock count down. The buzzer rang to my absolute relief.

I'd done it! I was World Champion in Italy, one of the toughest tournaments in the world! I was over the moon. As I lifted my trophy on the podium with the national anthem playing I beamed with pride because only ten years ago I was injecting Class A drugs at school. I'd fulfilled my dream.

I'm the Champion of the World.

AUTHOR BIO

WAYNE EVANS

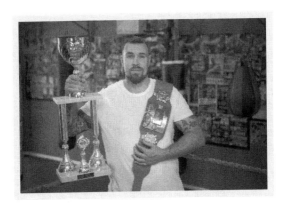

Wayne at thirty-seven years old has a vast amount of life experience under his belt. His experiences ranged from dealing with the deaths of loved ones at a young age, drugs, alcohol abuse, violence, dating a drug dealer at 16, locked up in a police cell, all whilst being raised by a single mother.

Wayne has turned his life around by becoming involved in kickboxing and is a born-again Christian, vowing to help people by setting up his own personal training business – helping over three hundred clients and running twenty-five successful boxing events in an eight-year period.

Wayne is now married to his wife Carrie and has two children, Isabel and Vivienne Rose, running a successful business to fulfil his purpose in life by touching as many lives as possible, all with the power of coaching and motivational speaking.

Qualifications:

Beginner/Intermediate/Advanced photography

Premiere Nutrition basics

GB Fitness Personal Trainer

NLP Practitioner

NLP Master Practitioner

Professional Life Coaching Diploma

Wayne specialises in changing lives with a combination of NLP techniques and one-to-one coaching.

He has helped clients beat depression, anxiety, suicidal thoughts and those stuck in a rut by setting new goals, finding the root cause of problems and changing careers.

He loves helping people with their personal development and believes it is one of the key ways to keep growing as a person.

Contact:

https://www.linkedin.com/in/wayne-evans-208ab652/

https://www.facebook.com/BOXFITPT

www.wayneevanscoaching.com

evanswayne@hotmail.com

facebook.com/WayneEvansDevelopmentCoach

instagram.com/wayne_evans82

31035666R00201

Printed in Great
Britain
by Amazon